# Orthodontics for the Craniofacial Surgery Patient

*Editors*

MICHAEL R. MARKIEWICZ
VEERASATHPURUSH ALLAREDDY
MICHAEL MILORO

## ORAL AND MAXILLOFACIAL SURGERY CLINICS OF NORTH AMERICA

www.oralmaxsurgery.theclinics.com

*Consulting Editor*
RUI P. FERNANDES

May 2020 • Volume 32 • Number 2

**ELSEVIER**

1600 John F. Kennedy Boulevard ● Suite 1800 ● Philadelphia, Pennsylvania, 19103-2899

http://www.oralmaxsurgery.theclinics.com

**ORAL AND MAXILLOFACIAL SURGERY CLINICS OF NORTH AMERICA Volume 32, Number 2**
**May 2020 ISSN 1042-3699, ISBN-13: 978-0-323-69492-6**

Editor: John Vassallo; j.vassallo@elsevier.com
Developmental Editor: Laura Fisher

*Oral and Maxillofacial Surgery Clinics of North America* (ISSN 1042-3699) is published quarterly by Elsevier Inc., 360 Park Avenue South, New York, NY 10010-1710. Months of issue are February, May, August, and November. Business and Editorial Offices: 1600 John F. Kennedy Blvd., Suite 1800, Philadelphia, PA 19103-2899. Periodicals postage paid at New York, NY and additional mailing offices. Subscription prices are $401.00 per year for US individuals, $756.00 per year for US institutions, $100.00 per year for US students/residents, $474.00 per year for Canadian individuals, $906.00 per year for Canadian institutions, $100.00 per year for Canadian students/residents, $525.00 per year for international individuals, $906.00 per year for international institutions and $235.00 per year for international students/residents. To receive student/resident rate, orders must be accompanied by name or affiliated institution, date of term, and the *signature* of program/residency coordinator on institution letterhead. Orders will be billed at individual rate until proof of status is received. Foreign air speed delivery is included in all *Clinics* subscription prices. All prices are subject to change without notice. **POSTMASTER:** Send address changes to *Oral and Maxillofacial Surgery Clinics of North America,* Elsevier Periodicals **Customer Service, 11830 Westline Industrial Drive, St. Louis, MO 63146. Tel: 1-800-654-2452 (U.S. and Canada); 314-447-8871 (outside U.S. and Canada). Fax: 314-447-8029. E-mail: journalscustomerservice-usa@elsevier.com (for print support); journalsonlinesupport-usa@elsevier.com (for online support).**

*Reprints.* For copies of 100 or more, of articles in this publication, please contact the Commercial Reprints Department, Elsevier Inc., 360 Park Avenue South, New York, NY 10010-1710. Tel.: 212-633-3874; Fax: 212-633-3820; Email: reprints@elsevier.com.

*Oral and Maxillofacial Surgery Clinics of North America* is covered in *MEDLINE/PubMed* (*Index Medicus*), *Science Citation Index Expanded (SciSearch®)*, *Journal Citation Reports/Science Edition*, and *Current Contents®/Clinical Medicine*.

# Contributors

## CONSULTING EDITOR

**RUI P. FERNANDES, MD, DMD, FACS, FRCS(Ed)**
Clinical Professor and Chief, Division of Head and Neck Surgery, Program Director, Head and Neck Oncologic Surgery and Microvascular Reconstruction Fellowship, Departments of Oral and Maxillofacial Surgery, Neurosurgery, and Orthopaedic Surgery and Rehabilitation, University of Florida Health Science Center, University of Florida College of Medicine, Jacksonville, Florida, USA

## EDITORS

**MICHAEL R. MARKIEWICZ, DDS MPH, MD, FACS**
Professor and Chair, Department of Oral and Maxillofacial Surgery, William M. Feagans Endowed Chair, Associate Dean for Hospital Affairs, School of Dental Medicine, Clinical Professor, Department of Neurosurgery, Division of Pediatric Surgery, Department of Surgery, Jacobs School of Medicine and Biomedical Sciences, University at Buffalo, Co-Director, Craniofacial Center of Western New York, John R. Oishei Children's Hospital, Buffalo, New York

**VEERASATHPURUSH ALLAREDDY, BDS, PhD**
Brodie Craniofacial Endowed Chair, Professor and Head, Department of Orthodontics, College of Dentistry, The University of Illinois at Chicago, Chicago, Illinois

**MICHAEL MILORO, DMD, MD, FACS**
Professor and Head, Department of Oral and Maxillofacial Surgery, College of Dentistry, The University of Illinois at Chicago, Chicago, Illinois

## AUTHORS

**VEERASATHPURUSH ALLAREDDY, BDS, PhD**
Brodie Craniofacial Endowed Chair, Professor and Head, Department of Orthodontics, College of Dentistry, The University of Illinois at Chicago, Chicago, Illinois

**SHAYNA AZOULAY-AVINOAM, DDS**
Resident, Department of Orthodontics, College of Dentistry, The University of Illinois at Chicago, Chicago, Illinois

**RICHARD BRUUN, DDS**
Craniofacial Orthodontist, Boston Children's Hospital, Cleft Lip/Palate and Craniofacial Teams, Assistant Professor of Developmental Biology, Part-Time, Harvard School of Dental Medicine, Senior Associate, Department of Dentistry, Boston Children's Hospital, Boston, Massachusetts, USA

**JENNIFER CAPLIN, DMD, MS**
Associate Director of Post Graduate Orthodontics, Assistant Professor, Department

of Orthodontics, College of Dentistry, The University of Illinois at Chicago, Chicago, Illinois

**STEPHANIE J. DREW, DMD, FACS**
Associate Professor, Department of Surgery, Division of Oral and Maxillofacial Surgery, Emory University School of Medicine, Atlanta, Georgia

**SEAN P. EDWARDS, DDS, MD**
Professor, Department of Oral and Maxillofacial Surgery, University of Michigan, Mott Children's Hospital, Ann Arbor, Michigan

**AUSTIN GAAL, DDS**
Former Cleft and Craniofacial Fellow, The University of Oklahoma, College of Dentistry, Department of Oral and Maxillofacial Surgery, Oklahoma University Children's Hospital, JW Keys Cleft and Craniofacial Clinic, Oklahoma City, Oklahoma, USA; Cascadia OMS, Kirkland, Washington, USA

**GHALI E. GHALI, DDS, MD, FACS, FRCS(Ed)**
Jack W. Gamble Professor and Chairman, Department of Oral and Maxillofacial Surgery/ Head and Neck Surgery, Chancellor, Louisiana State University Health Sciences Center, Shreveport, Louisiana

**JEFFREY HAMMOUDEH, DDS, MD**
Associate Chief Plastic and Maxillofacial Surgery, Associate Professor, University of Southern California, Division of Oral and Maxillofacial Surgery, Department of Plastic and Reconstructive Surgery, Children's Hospital Los Angeles, Los Angeles, California

**RICHARD A. HOPPER, MD, MS**
Chief, Pediatric Plastic and Craniofacial Surgery, Marlys C. Larson Professor of Craniofacial Surgery, University of Washington School of Medicine, Craniofacial Center, Division of Plastic and Craniofacial Surgery, Seattle Children's Hospital, Seattle, Washington

**HITESH KAPADIA, DDS, PhD**
Chief, Division of Craniofacial Orthodontics, Seattle Children's Hospital, Craniofacial Center, Seattle, Washington

**JAMES MacLAINE, BDS**
Clinical Instructor, Department of Developmental Biology, Boston Children's Hospital, Harvard School of Dental Medicine, Boston, Massachusetts

**ASHLEY E. MANLOVE, DMD, MD**
Clinical Instructor, Program Director, Director of Carle Cleft and Craniofacial Team, Department of Oral and Maxillofacial Surgery, Carle Foundation Hospital, Urbana, Illinois

**MICHAEL R. MARKIEWICZ, DDS MPH, MD, FACS**
Professor and Chair, Department of Oral and Maxillofacial Surgery, William M. Feagans Endowed Chair, Associate Dean for Hospital Affairs, School of Dental Medicine, Clinical Professor, Department of Neurosurgery, Division of Pediatric Surgery, Department of Surgery, Jacobs School of Medicine and Biomedical Sciences, University at Buffalo, Co-Director, Craniofacial Center of Western New York, John R. Oishei Children's Hospital, Buffalo, New York

**MARK A. MILLER, MD, DMD**
Assistant Professor, Departments of Oral and Maxillofacial Surgery, Neurosurgery, and Pediatrics, UT Health San Antonio, San Antonio, Texas

**DOUGLAS OLSON, DMD, MS**
Craniofacial Center of Western New York, Oishei Children's Outpatient Center, Buffalo, New York

**BONNIE L. PADWA, DMD, MD**
Oral Surgeon-in-Chief, Section of Oral and Maxillofacial Surgery, Associate Professor, Department of Plastic and Oral Surgery, Harvard Medical School, Boston, Massachusetts

**VICTORIA PALERMO, MD, DDS**
Florida Craniofacial Institute, Tampa, Florida

**YASSMIN PARSAEI, DMD**
Orthodontic Resident, Division of Orthodontics, Department of Craniofacial Sciences, University of Connecticut, Farmington, Connecticut

**STAVAN Y. PATEL, DDS, MD**
Assistant Professor and Residency Program Director, Department of Oral and Maxillofacial Surgery/Head and Neck Surgery, Louisiana State University Health Sciences Center, Shreveport, Louisiana

**JEFFREY C. POSNICK, DMD, MD**
Professor Emeritus, Plastic and Reconstructive Surgery and Pediatrics, Georgetown University, Washington, DC; Professor of Orthodontics, University of Maryland, Baltimore College of Dental Surgery, Baltimore, Maryland; Professor of Oral and Maxillofacial Surgery, Howard University College of Dentistry, Washington, DC

**CORY M. RESNICK, DMD, MD**
Attending Physician, Oral and Maxillofacial Surgery Program, Assistant Professor, Department of Plastic and Oral Surgery, Harvard Medical School, Boston, Massachusetts

**PAT RICALDE, MD, DDS**
Director, Florida Craniofacial Institute, St. Joseph's Cleft and Craniofacial Center, Tampa, Florida

**GERARDO ROMEO, DDS, MD, MBA**
Division Chief and Program Director, Oral and Maxillofacial Surgery, Departments of Dental Medicine, and Pediatrics, Northwell Health, Medical Co-Director, Hagedorn Cleft and Craniofacial Team at Cohen Children's Medical Center, Assistant Professor, Donald and Barbara Zucker School of Medicine at Hofstra/Northwell, Long Island Jewish Medical Center, New Hyde Park, New York

**ELIZABETH ROSS, DDS**
Clinical Instructor, Department of Developmental Biology, Boston Children's Hospital, Harvard School of Dental Medicine, Boston, Massachusetts

**RAMON RUIZ, DMD, MD**
Arnold Palmer Hospital for Children, Orlando, Florida

**CURTIS D. SCHMIDT, DDS**
Cleft and Craniofacial Surgery Fellow, Department of Oral and Maxillofacial Surgery/

Head and Neck Surgery, Louisiana State University Health Sciences Center, Shreveport, Louisiana

**STEPHEN SHUSTERMAN, DMD**
Clinical Associate Professor, Harvard School of Dental Medicine, Dentist-in-Chief, Emeritus, Boston Children's Hospital, Boston, Massachusetts

**KEVIN S. SMITH, DDS, FACS, FACD**
Professor and Resident/Fellowship Program Director, The University of Oklahoma, College of Dentistry, Department of Oral and Maxillofacial Surgery, Director, JW Keys Cleft and Craniofacial Clinic, Children's Hospital of Oklahoma, University of Tulsa, MK Chapman Cleft and Craniofacial Clinic, Profiles Oral Facial Surgery Experts, Oklahoma City, Oklahoma, USA

**DEREK STEINBACHER, MD, DMD, FACS**
Chief of Oral and Maxillofacial Surgery, Director of Craniofacial Surgery, Associate Professor, Section of Plastic and Reconstructive Surgery, Yale School of Medicine, New Haven, Connecticut

**SRINIVAS M. SUSARLA, DMD, MD, MPH**
Assistant Professor of Surgery (Plastic), University of Washington School of Medicine, Assistant Professor of Oral-Maxillofacial Surgery, University of Washington School of Dentistry, Craniofacial Center, Divisions of Craniofacial and Plastic Surgery and Oral-Maxillofacial Surgery, Seattle Children's Hospital, Seattle, Washington

**TIMOTHY J. TREMONT, DMD, MS**
Professor and Chairman, Department of Orthodontics, Medical University of South Carolina, Charleston, South Carolina

**RAYMOND TSE, MD**
Seattle Children's Hospital, Craniofacial Center, Seattle, Washington

**MARK URATA, DDS, MD, FACS**
Audrey Skirball Kenis Endowed Chair and Chief, Division of Plastic Surgery and reconstructive Maxillofacial Surgery, Chair

Division of Oral and Maxillofacial Surgery, Ostrow School of Dentistry, University of Southern California, Children's Hospital Los Angeles, Los Angeles, California

**FLAVIO URIBE, DDS, MDentSc**
Charles Burstone Professor, Program Director and Interim Chair, Division of Orthodontics, Department of Craniofacial Sciences, University of Connecticut, Farmington, Connecticut

**SHANKAR RENGASAMY VENUGOPALAN, DDS, DMSc, CAGE (Ortho), PhD**
Department of Orthodontics, Associate Professor, The University of Iowa, College of Dentistry and Dental Clinics, Iowa City, Iowa

**JENNIFER E. WOERNER, DMD, MD, FACS**
Assistant Professor and Fellowship Director, Cleft and Craniofacial Surgery, Department of Oral and Maxillofacial Surgery/Head and Neck Surgery, Louisiana State University Health Sciences Center, Shreveport, Louisiana

**SUMIT YADAV, MDS, PhD**
Associate Professor, Department of Craniofacial Sciences, University of Connecticut School of Dental Medicine, Farmington, Connecticut

**DAVID YATES, DMD, MD, FACS**
Program Director, EPCH Cleft and Craniofacial Fellowship, Division Chief of Cranial and Facial Surgery, El Paso Children's Hospital, Clinical Assistant Professor of Surgery, Texas Tech University Health Sciences Center El Paso, Paul L. Foster School of Medicine, Partner, High Desert Oral & Facial Surgery, El Paso, Texas

**STEPHEN YEN, DMD, PhD**
Director of Fellowship in Craniofacial and Special Needs Orthodontics, Division of Dentistry, Children's Hospital Los Angeles, Center for Craniofacial Molecular Biology, University of Southern California, Los Angeles, California

# Contents

lip elements, the lower lateral cartilages, and the columella achieved with NAM are helpful for creating a suitable platform for tension-free lip repair.

This article provides an overview of the orthodontic preparation prior to secondary alveolar bone grafting of alveolar defects in those with complete cleft lip and palate. Use of cone beam computed tomography in diagnosis and treatment planning for addressing alveolar clefts, the rationale for maxillary expansion prior to alveolar bone grafting, key steps in differential maxillary expansion, potential adverse effects, and outcomes associated with maxillary expansion are provided in this overview.

Reconstruction of large craniofacial defects requires several factors to be considered before deciding on the best reconstructive option. This article discusses various factors taken into consideration when deciding on which reconstructive option is ideal for a given patient and defect. For large craniofacial defects, reconstruction using tissue transfer is considered preferentially over obturation, although in select defects obturation using a traditional tooth- or implant-borne prosthetic obturator can be considered a viable option.

This article provides an overview of epidemiology, genetics, and common orofacial features of those with craniosynostosis. Patients with craniosynostosis require several surgical procedures along with continuum of care. The earliest surgical interventions are done during the first few years of life to relieve the fused sutures. Midface advancement, limited phase of orthodontic treatment, and combined orthodontics/orthognathic surgery treatment are usually required during later years. This article presents several examples of cases with outcomes associated with these procedures.

Preparation and planning for orthognathic surgery in late adolescence depends on the complexity of unresolved problems with which the patient presents. Different strategies are presented to address these unresolved problems in the adult patient with cleft lip and palate. Different surgical and orthodontic treatments are presented to correct the class III malocclusion in patients with cleft lip and palate in ranges that are analogous to the envelope of discrepancy. For complex cases, the principles of achievability, stability, and esthetics should guide the decision-making process for planning the preparation for orthognathic surgery.

## LeFort Distraction in the Cleft Patient

Stephanie J. Drew and Hitesh Kapadia

The cleft patient may present with significant maxillary deficiency requiring maxillary advancement to establish balanced facial form and function. Often these skeletal advancements require movement of the maxilla of more than 10 mm. The cleft patient poses special challenges because of difficulty of mobilizing tissues on a multiply operated maxilla, as well as long-term stability. Distraction osteogenesis is a technique that may be applied to help move the maxilla over a long distance and slowly expand the soft tissues. A discussion of the orthodontic and surgical considerations when planning and executing the technique is presented.

## Orthodontic and Surgical Principles for Distraction Osteogenesis in Children with Pierre-Robin Sequence

Stephen Yen, Austin Gaal, and Kevin Smith

Patients with Pierre-Robin sequence recalcitrant to nonsurgical intervention have historically required tracheostomy. Mandibular distraction provides a predictable alternative treatment to tracheostomy for improving airway. Orthodontic perioperative interventions should be considered, including overcorrection, placement of temporary anchorage devices, elastics, and molding the regenerate. Mandibular distraction can be technically difficult and may cause complications. Performed correctly, mandibular distraction provides patients with a better quality of life than tracheostomy.

## Orthodontics for Unilateral and Bilateral Cleft Deformities

Yassmin Parsaei, Flavio Uribe, and Derek Steinbacher

Orthodontic treatment of patients with unilateral and bilateral cleft palate requires an extensive interdisciplinary approach to achieve optimal functional and esthetic rehabilitation. Intervention is divided into 3 main stages: early mixed, late mixed, and permanent dentition. Treatment modalities can vary according to developmental stage, severity of cleft, and presence of other dentofacial abnormalities. This article describes the use and efficacy of different orthodontic, orthopedic, and surgical approaches at each developmental stage of unilateral and bilateral clefts, whereby the orthodontist plays a pivotal role in the different phases of growth and development of the cleft lip and the patient.

## Surgical-Orthodontic Considerations in Subcranial and Frontofacial Distraction

Richard A. Hopper, Hitesh Kapadia, and Srinivas M. Susarla

Subcranial and frontofacial distraction osteogenesis have emerged as powerful tools for management of hypoplasia involving the upper two-thirds of the face. The primary goal of subcranial or frontofacial distraction is to improve the orientation of the upper face and midface structures (frontal bone, orbitozygomatic complex, maxilla, nasal complex) relative to the cranial base, globes, and mandible. The various techniques used are tailored for management of specific phenotypic differences in facial position and may include segmental osteotomies, differential vectors, or synchronous maxillomandibular rotation.

An understanding of fundamental orthodontic principles involving diagnosis, treatment planning, and clinical strategies is essential for achieving successful outcomes in the treatment of craniofacial patients, particularly cleft lip/palate. This article focuses on: customizing a mandibular dental arch form using the WALA ridge; accurately diagnosing the maxillary skeletal transverse dimension (cusp to cusp/fossa to fossa); coordinating the upper dental arch with the lower; using a smiling profile and glabella vertical to assess anteroposterior jaw position; and leveling the mandibular curve of Spee while considering the lower one-third of the face. These concepts influence treatment outcomes to the extent they are used.

# ORAL AND MAXILLOFACIAL SURGERY CLINICS OF NORTH AMERICA

## FORTHCOMING ISSUES

*August 2020*
**Global Oral and Maxillofacial Surgery**
Shahid R. Aziz, Jose M. Marchena, and Steven M. Roser, *Editors*

*November 2020*
**Dentoalveolar Surgery**
Somsak Sittitavornwong, *Editor*

*February 2021*
**Modern Rhinoplasty and the Management of its Complications**
Shahrokh C. Bagheri, Husain Ali Khan, and Behnam Bohluli, *Editors*

## RECENT ISSUES

*February 2020*
**Orthodontics for the Oral and Maxillofacial Surgery Patient**
Michael R. Markiewicz, Veerasathpurush Allareddy, and Michael Miloro, *Editors*

*November 2019*
**Advances in Oral and Maxillofacial Surgery**
Jose M. Marchena, Jonathan W. Shum, and Jonathon S. Jundt, *Editors*

*August 2019*
**Dental Implants, Part II: Computer Technology**
Ole T. Jensen, *Editor*

---

### SERIES OF RELATED INTEREST

*Atlas of the Oral and Maxillofacial Surgery Clinics*
www.oralmaxsurgeryatlas.theclinics.com

*Dental Clinics*
www.dental.theclinics.com

---

**THE CLINICS ARE NOW AVAILABLE ONLINE!**
Access your subscription at:
**www.theclinics.com**

# Preface
# Orthodontics for the Craniofacial Surgery Patient

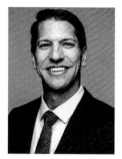
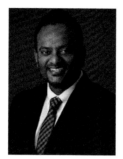
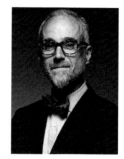

Michael R. Markiewicz, DDS,
MPH, MD, FACS

Veerasathpurush Allareddy,
BDS, PhD

Michael Miloro, DMD, MD, FACS

*Editors*

This issue of the *Oral and Maxillofacial Surgery Clinics of North America* serves as the second of a 2-part series that emphasizes the critical role of the orthodontist in the management of the craniofacial surgery patient (issue 2). The first issue, "Orthodontics for the Oral and Maxillofacial Surgery Patient" (issue 1), reviewed, in detail, common collaborative procedures performed by the orthodontist and oral and maxillofacial surgeon as viewed from the joint and integrated perspectives of both specialties. This issue, "Orthodontics for the Craniofacial Surgery Patient," highlights the critical role that the orthodontist plays in the surgical procedures performed for the craniofacial patient.

The impetus for this work was initiated with the goal of developing a comprehensive reference text describing the most commonly performed procedures involving craniofacial surgeons and craniofacial orthodontists by experienced authors in both specialties. The editors feel that this was an often-overlooked area in the existing literature. To address this goal, as in the first issue in this series, we again feel that we have been so fortunate to recruit some of the most notable craniofacial surgeons and craniofacial orthodontists in the world to write on topics and share their experiences for which they are considered authoritative experts. We are very proud of this text and so grateful to those who have contributed to making this a unique collaboration of practitioners.

As in the first issue of this series, we charged authors (oral and maxillofacial surgeons and orthodontists) with the task of collaboration based upon their expertise, regardless of their institution or prior interactions or biases. A significant challenge in achieving this goal, and major difficulty for these authors, is that they may not have ever met each other. Yet they were still able to work together and produce quality articles for this text. All the authors, regardless of institutional and preconceived biases, agreed to join us on this monumental endeavor. Each of the authors produced a thoughtful and authoritative article for the topic for which they were assigned, and we, the editors, are so thankful for this.

Finally, these patients described in this issue are so special to us, and we are fortunate enough to be able to treat them and make meaningful changes in their lives. They are unique, complex, challenging, and perplexing, often requiring us to "think outside the box." Perhaps most importantly, treating these patients is truly rewarding and an honor for us all. We hope this text will help to

Oral Maxillofacial Surg Clin N Am 32 (2020) xiii–xiv
https://doi.org/10.1016/j.coms.2020.02.001
1042-3699/20/© 2020 Published by Elsevier Inc.

contribute positively to their care by reinforcing the critical relationships between specialists in achieving successful outcomes.

Michael R. Markiewicz, DDS, MPH, MD, FACS
Department of Oral and Maxillofacial Surgery
School of Dental Medicine
University at Buffalo
3435 Main Street, 112 Squire Hall
Buffalo, NY 14214, USA

Department of Neurosurgery
Division of Pediatric Surgery
Department of Surgery
Jacobs School of Medicine and Biomedical
Sciences

Craniofacial Center of Western New York
John R. Oishei Children's Hospital
Buffalo, NY, USA

Veerasathpurush Allareddy, BDS, PhD
Department of Orthodontics
College of Dentistry
University of Illinois at Chicago
801 South Paulina Street
138AD (MC841)
Chicago, IL 60612-7211, USA

Michael Miloro, DMD, MD, FACS
Department of Oral and Maxillofacial Surgery
College of Dentistry
University of Illinois at Chicago
801 South Paulina Street
M/C 835
Chicago, IL 60612-7211, USA

*E-mail addresses:*
mrm25@buffalo.edu (M.R. Markiewicz)
sath@uic.edu (V. Allareddy)
mmiloro@uic.edu (M. Miloro)

# Craniofacial Growth: Current Theories and Influence on Management

Ashley E. Manlove, DMD, MD[a], Gerardo Romeo, DDS, MD, MBA[b,c],
Shankar Rengasamy Venugopalan, DDS, DMSc, CAGE (Ortho), PhD[d,*]

## KEYWORDS

- Craniofacial growth • Maxillofacial growth/development • Facial growth/development
- Dentofacial growth/development • Craniofacial development • Craniomaxillofacial surgery
- Orthodontics

## KEY POINTS

- To maximize outcomes and minimize iatrogenic consequences to growth, a strong foundational knowledge of craniofacial growth is a requirement of any practitioner.
- There is a cephalo-caudal gradient of growth potential during craniofacial growth.
- The development of the craniofacial skeleton occurs as a result of a sequence of normal developmental events.

## INTRODUCTION

The management of craniofacial abnormalities and associated malocclusion requires well-coordinated collaborative efforts from several specialists. The impact of growth of the craniofacial skeleton on successful treatment cannot be understated. To maximize outcomes and minimize iatrogenic consequences to growth, a strong foundational knowledge of craniofacial growth is a requirement of any practitioner. Proper sequencing and timing of interventions are critical in optimizing outcomes. At times, interventions that are harmful are avoided until the preservation of growth allows for it (ie, secondary alveolar cleft bone grafting in contrast to primary) and other times, interventions are used to manipulate growth to either increase or limit it (ie, orthodontic head gear and cranial orthotics).

Despite a long history of study and strong supportive evidence for certain theories, no single theory, to date, appears to completely capture all aspects of craniofacial growth. With various theories in existence, genetic control theory and functional matrix theory are the 2 most popular and widely accepted. It is highly likely that some amalgamation of various theories would be close to true description of the concepts of craniofacial growth. This article reviews some basic terminologies of growth and development, core concepts of normal growth, components of craniofacial growth, growth by tissue types and anatomic subunits, and growth modification by orthodontic intervention.

## BASIC TERMINOLOGY

The terms "development" and "growth" are related to one another and typically discussed in

[a] Department of Oral and Maxillofacial Surgery, Carle Cleft and Craniofacial Team, Carle Foundation Hospital, 611 W. Park Street, Urbana, IL 61801, USA; [b] Oral and Maxillofacial Surgery, Department of Dental Medicine, Northwell Health, Hagedorn Cleft and Craniofacial Team at Cohen Children's Medical Center, Hofstra Northwell School of Medicine, Long Island Jewish Medical Center, 270–05 76th Avenue, New Hyde Park, NY 11040, USA; [c] Department of Pediatrics, Northwell Health, Hagedorn Cleft and Craniofacial Team at Cohen Children's Medical Center, Hofstra Northwell School of Medicine, New Hyde Park, NY, USA; [d] Department of Orthodontics, The University of Iowa, College of Dentistry and Dental Clinics, 801 Newton Road, DSB, S232, Iowa City, IA 52242, USA
* Corresponding author.
E-mail address: Shankar-Venugopalan@uiowa.edu

Oral Maxillofacial Surg Clin N Am 32 (2020) 167–175
https://doi.org/10.1016/j.coms.2020.01.007
1042-3699/20/© 2020 Elsevier Inc. All rights reserved.

tandem or even interchangeably. Conceptually, however, they are distinct. The term "development" describes formation, differentiation, or specialization of tissues/subunits, usually by transitioning in anatomic form. On the contrary, the term "growth" refers to increase in size of any tissue, subunit, or unit.

Craniofacial development and growth begin in utero and continue variably into adulthood. Three main parameters are typically used to describe "growth" in the literature: *magnitude*, *direction,* and *velocity*. The "magnitude" is used to categorize growth in terms of some "relative amount" for a given dimension (transverse, sagittal, and vertical). The "direction," however, is typically simplified into a vector representing the "net" directional growth. The term "velocity" refers to the rate of growth per unit time.

It is common to hear the term "skeletal maturity" used when planning interventions among practitioners. Often times, skeletal maturity determines whether or not an intervention is deemed to be indicated or contraindicated. Although some would mistakenly assume that "maturity" is cessation of growth, a more accurate interpretation of "maturity" would connote most of the magnitude and peak velocity of growth has occurred.

## CORE CONCEPTS OF NORMAL GROWTH AND DEVELOPMENT
### Concept 1

All individuals go through similar stages of development and growth, albeit not always to the same extent or at the exact same time.[1] The chronologic age, skeletal age, and dental age do not always correlate in an individual. Conception to birth averages 40 weeks and is termed the "prenatal" period. Development and growth in terms of magnitude and velocity are highest in the prenatal period. From birth to 2 years (infancy), the magnitude and velocity of growth and development decreases until it plateaus in childhood. During puberty, the magnitude and velocity of growth increases again. Following pubertal growth, the magnitude and velocity of growth steadily decreases.

### Concept 2

Not all tissue types or parts of the body grow at the same time or the same rate. In the craniofacial subunits, not only are various tissue types present, but those tissues are present in variable proportions at different times during growth and development. For example, in a given time point, the growth for neural or lymphoid tissues are different in magnitude and velocity than, say, any single bone of the facial skeleton.

### Concept 3

Growth potential is driven by genetics and influenced by environmental factors. "Normal growth" occurs on a spectrum of what would be considered "normal." There are varying degrees of deviation from what would be considered a normal craniofacial and dentofacial relationship, which are determined by the inherent genetic makeup. Those genetic predispositions, however, are subject to environmental influences. At the macro level, growth potential of all tissues and subunits can only be realized if physiology is unimpeded by pathology (ie, proper nutrition and absence of disease). At the micro level, introduction of an unfavorable variable (ie, surgical scarring) on a growing tissue type or subunit can also negatively impact the achievement of the genetically programmed growth potential. Some tissues are more susceptible to environmental influence than others.

## CRANIOFACIAL GROWTH BY TISSUE TYPE

In the craniofacial region, growth of different tissue types, anatomic units, and functional spaces occur in a coordinated relationship to one another at different rates and time points (**Fig. 1**). It is widely accepted that complex signaling between these tissue types and anatomic units must occur in a precise fashion to achieve normal growth both in utero and throughout life. The major components of the craniofacial growth are neural tissue, muscle, tonsils/adenoids, cartilage, bone, sutures, and functioning spaces.

### Neural Tissue

Neural tissue completes much of its growth early in development. At birth, the neural tissues have achieved approximately 60% to 70% of adult size. By early childhood, neural tissues reach 95% of adult dimensions. The growth of neural tissues (brain and globes) drives the growth of the surrounding bone and musculoskeletal tissues around them. Functional matrix hypothesis, as described by Moss and Salentijn,[2] postulates that it is the soft tissue growth (the brain and soft tissue envelope) that induces bone and sutural growth of the cranium.

### Muscle

The muscle tissue of the craniofacial region is less than 50% of adult size at birth. By the time neural tissues have reached maturity, muscle tissue has

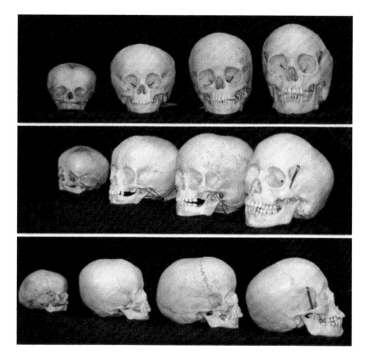

**Fig. 1.** Multiple views of skulls from infancy through adolescence show the progression of craniofacial bone growth. The general progression is from superior to inferior with a downward and forward growth vector. (*From* Costello BJ, Mooney MP, Shand JM. Craniomaxillofacial surgery in the pediatric patient: growth and development considerations. In: Fonseca RJ, editor. Oral and maxillofacial surgery. 3rd ed. St. Louis: Elsevier; 2018. p. 627-44; with permission.)

reached only approximately 70% of adult dimensions in the craniofacial region. Muscle dimensions develop later in childhood and adolescence to support the adult dentition, skeletal frame, phonation, and deglutition. The muscles are considered adaptive in nature and grow to support function.[2]

### Tonsils/Adenoids

Lymphoid tissues actually exceed adult size in childhood. The dimensions of the tonsils and adenoids are approximately 125% of adult size by age 5. The lymphoid tissues regress in size after 5 years of age and are in part responsible for further development of the functional pharyngeal space. This involution of lymphoid tissue must be taken into consideration, particularly, in patients with cleft palate, as it can result in worsening of velopharyngeal dysfunction as the child gets older.[3]

### Cartilage and Chondrogenesis

During early development, there are 2 kinds of cartilage: (1) primary and (2) secondary. The primary cartilage is unique in that it grows interstitially, it is pressure tolerant (as compared with bone, for example), and is nonvascular in nature. Work by Scott[4] postulates that primary cartilage is genetically driven and acts as a growth center driving much of the net change in craniofacial form during development. The cranial base and

nasal septum are derived from primary cartilage. The growth of the nasomaxillary complex is dictated by the growth of the cranial base and nasal septal cartilage. Most primary cartilage of the cranial base is replaced by bone via endochondral ossification early in childhood thus primary cartilage as a "driver of growth" ends relatively early.[4] On the contrary, the secondary cartilage is not under genetic control in the same way as primary cartilage. It is considered more "adaptive in nature" in that it does grow and ultimately ossify, but it does so in response to function and is under significant environmental influence. In the craniofacial skeleton, secondary cartilage is found in the condylar head, coronoid process, angle of the mandible, and mental protuberance.

### Bone and Osteogenesis

Bone is a calcified tissue, which is highly vascular, sensitive to pressure, and is subjected to environmental influences.[5] The bone formation during development occurs by either intramembranous or endochondral ossification. During intramembranous ossification, the mesenchymal cells differentiate directly to osteogenic cells, whereas in endochondral ossification, cartilage serves as a template, which is then replaced by bone. Overall bone growth does not occur due to surface apposition of bone. Rather, the bone growth occurs by

2 major mechanisms: (1) cortical drift: periosteal deposition of bone and endosteal resorption of bone; and (2) displacement: physical movement of bone due to growth of the adjacent structure.[5] It must be remembered that bone growth is not static, rather dynamic. Even after reaching adult dimensions, bone undergoes near constant remodeling. Furthermore, the periosteum that surrounds the bone has a powerful influence over its growth and development. Therefore, interruption of that periosteum has the potential to affect the growth potential of the bone.[3]

## Sutures

The cranial sutures are fibrous articulations formed between the approximating osteogenic fronts of the bones of cranial vault. On the external surface of the suture lies the fibrous layer of periosteum and on the internal surface lies the fibrous layer of dura mater. In-between the approximating osteogenic fronts of the suture lies the mesenchyme, which provides a source for new osteogenic cells.[6] The sutures are important sites of compensatory growth and play an important role in craniofacial growth.[7] The growth at sutures occurs as an adaptation to the growth of the neural tissue and surrounding tissues such as primary cartilage or soft tissue. New bone is deposited incrementally across those sutures with remodeling and displacement occurring in a harmonious physiologic balance under normal circumstances[8]

## Functioning Spaces

As described by Moss and Salentijn,[2] the craniofacial region contains various spaces that support function, for example, respiration, deglutition, vision, olfaction, and cognition/neural integration. The different tissue types grow in support of said functions resulting in "functioning spaces." An example would be that although neural integration is the most essential of craniofacial functions, growth of the brain occurs early and quickly. The growth of the brain in turn drives growth of the cranium. Another example would be that after birth, alimentation becomes a higher-order function, therefore swallowing and jaw movement drive the development of the functioning oral cavity and growth of bone, teeth, and muscle to support that function. Enlow and colleagues[5,9] described 2 main morphologic events that direct craniofacial growth, including (1) growth of the basal cranium, and (2) development of pharyngeal and facial airway structures. According to his theory, remodeling occurs as compensatory changes of tissue to adapt to function, as described by the functional matrix hypothesis of Moss and Salentijn.[2]

## CRANIOFACIAL GROWTH BY ANATOMIC SUBUNIT
### Cranium

The cranial vault and the cranial base make up the entire cranium. The cranial vault is composed of intramembranously formed bones, where bone growth occurs at the fibrous suture articulations. The cranial vault grows exponentially during the first year of life, reaching approximately 86% of its adult size by 1 year of age and 94% of adult size by 5 years of age.[10] This reflects the significant neurodevelopment that occurs during this timeframe. A practical application of this knowledge is the orthotic treatment of positional plagiocephaly has become more prevalent with the "back to sleep" campaign. As parents are instructed to place their infants on their back when sleeping, this can cause flattening of the occiput and compensatory frontal bossing. Newborns lack the neuromuscular strength and control of neck muscles during this exponential neurodevelopment and rapid growth of their cranial vault, which can lead to significant flattening and dysmorphic cranial vault growth. Given that most cranial vault growth occurs during the first year of life, cranial orthotic therapy is most effective from 4 months of age until 1 year of age.

Contrary to the cranial vault, the cranial base is composed of bones that form by endochondral ossification. By 5 years of age the anterior cranial base is more matured (~90% of adult size) compared with the posterior cranial base (80% of adult size). The cranial base growth occurs interstitially at articulations called synchondroses, a major growth center in the craniofacial skeleton. There are 3 synchondroses at the cranial base: (1) intersphenoidal synchondroses, which fuse at the time of birth; (2) sphenoethmoidal synchondroses, which fuse at ~7 to 8 years of age; and (3) sphenooccipital synchondroses, which fuse shortly after puberty. Cranial growth discrepancy also can occur from craniosynostosis, which is the premature fusion of cranial vault sutures. Single-suture craniosynostosis is most common and usually nonsyndromic.[11] Multisuture craniosynostosis can occur and is more common in conditions such as Apert, Pfeiffer, Crouzon, and Saethre-Chotzen syndromes. Treatment of cranial growth discrepancy from premature fusion of cranial sutures is usually performed at approximately 10 months of age as cranial growth is slowing down, but surgery will still allow for appropriate volume for brain growth to occur. Cessation of cranial growth occurs at 14 years of age for girls and 15 years of age for boys.

## Orbits

The orbit is composed of bones from the naso-maxillary complex (palatine, maxillary, zygomatic bones), as well as from the cranial vault (frontal, ethmoid, sphenoid, lacrimal bones). The growth in this region occurs at the sutures between these bones. Orbital growth occurs rapidly in the first year of life in association with the growth of the cranial base, vault, and globes. Most orbital bone growth is complete at approximately 5 years of age.[12,13] Intercanthal width is complete at 8 years of age in girls and 11 years of age in boys. Orbital height growth is more gradual when compared with orbital volume, which ultimately contributes to midfacial height. Disruption of normal orbital growth is seen in unicoronal craniosynostosis (**Fig. 2**), as well as in Tessier clefts (**Fig. 3**) that involve any of the bones that construct the orbit.

## Nose

An infant's nose has more cartilage than bone when compared with an adult nose. There are 2 main periods of growth of the nose: 2 to 5 years of age and then during puberty. The septal cartilage is thought to be a major growth center and driving force in midface growth early in development. The perpendicular plate arises from endochondral ossification along the skull base and eventually meets with the vomer at approximately 6 to 8 years of age through cartilage growth and ossification.[14] In addition, where the vomer and premaxilla meet is an important growth center. This suture line is abnormal in cleft patients and may contribute to asymmetric nasal growth in the cleft population.[15]

## Zygoma

The zygomatic bones also grow quickly during the first year of life with cessation of growth at approximately 5 to 7 years of age. By 5 years of age the bizygomatic width is 83% of adult width and the width of the face is mature at 13 years of age in girls and 15 years of age in boys.[12,13] Zygomatic deformities can be seen following trauma as well as in congenital disorders such as Treacher Collins and craniofacial dysostosis.

## Maxilla

The maxilla develops by intramembranous ossification. The growth at the cranial base exerts a major influence on maxillary growth, resulting in a downward and forward displacement. In a compensatory fashion to this displacement, bone is deposited at the circumaxillary and intermaxillary sutures, and resorbed from the anterior surface of the maxilla. In addition, maxillary growth is also dependent on early nasal septal growth. In the antero-posterior direction, bone is deposited in the maxillary tuberosity region, which contributes to the lengthening of the maxilla to accommodate developing dentition. Furthermore, as the maxilla descends during growth, bone is resorbed from the nasal floor and deposited in the palatal vault.

The premaxillary/maxillary suture fuses at approximately 3 to 5 years of age, the midpalatal suture fuses at approximately 15 to 18 years of age, and the transpalatal suture fuses at approximately 20 to 25 years of age.[16–18] The vertical height of the maxilla reaches its maximum growth at approximately 12 years of age in girls and 15 years of age in boys.[12,13] The anterior projection of the maxilla reaches skeletal maturity at

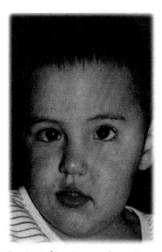
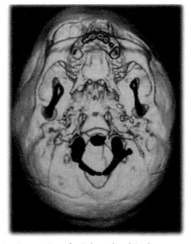
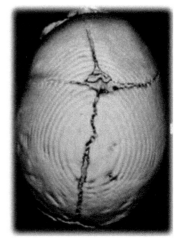

**Fig. 2.** Left unicoronal craniosynostosis causing facial and orbital asymmetry.

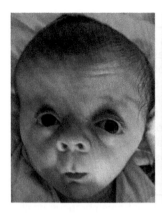
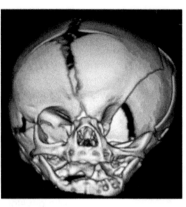

**Fig. 3.** Tessier orbital cleft 9 to 10 in conjunction with left unicoronal craniosynostosis causing significant dysmorphia and facial asymmetry.

13 years of age in girls and 14 years of age in boys. Growth and development of the maxilla parallels growth and pneumatization of the maxillary sinus. Midface hypoplasia is a clinical phenotype in patients with achondroplasia, craniofacial dysostosis syndromes, as an iatrogenic effect in patients with cleft lip/palate, and as a result of trauma in midface and nasal fractures.[19]

## Mandible

The body of the mandible develops by intramembranous ossification and the condyle by endochondral ossification. In the craniofacial complex, the mandible has the greatest postnatal growth potential. With reference to the cranial base, the mandible is displaced downward and forward; however, the direction of growth at the condyle, a major contributor of postnatal growth, is upward and backward. During growth, increase in the corpus length is achieved by resorption along the anterior surface of the ramus and deposition along the posterior surface of the ramus. Furthermore, the mandibular width increases by bone deposition along the buccal surface. Therefore, growth of the mandible occurs in all regions, including the condyles, rami, and body through displacement and remodeling.[5,20]

Mandibular width is nearly complete at 5 years of age. Mandibular height reaches maturity at 12 years in girls and 15 years in boys. Mandibular anterior projection growth is complete at 13 years of age in girls and 15 years of age in boys.[12,13] Mandibular hypoplasia is commonly seen in Pierre Robin sequence, craniofacial microsomia, Treacher Collins syndrome, Nager syndrome, condylar trauma, and idiopathic condylar resorption, among other causes. Mandibular hyperplasia can be genetic and is also seen in acromegaly.

## Tooth Formation and Eruption

The process of tooth formation is under tight genetic control and takes place by reciprocal interaction between the dental epithelium and neural crest derived mesenchyme.[21] The development and eruption of the dentition is closely intertwined with growth and development of the maxilla and mandible. Development of the primary dentition is initiated by the sixth week of gestation, and the permanent dentition is initiated at approximately the 10th to 13th week.[21] In a normal-growing patient, all primary teeth are erupted in the maxilla and mandible by 2 to 2.5 years of age. All permanent teeth except third molars erupt by 12 to 13 years of age. This is routinely delayed in patients with cleft. For teeth to erupt, dental follicles initiate resorption of bone along the path of eruption and bone is deposited on the opposite end.[22] Most teeth emerge when half to two-thirds of root is formed and the root formation is fully complete by 2 to 4 years after eruption. There is therefore a net increase in the bone that supports teeth that is associated with eruption.

Tooth eruption is rather a dynamic process and the rate of eruption parallels the rate of jaw growth. During adolescence, the maxillary and mandibular molars drift mesially by ~0.6 mm per year and ~0.5 mm per year, respectively,[23] whereas the maxillary and mandibular incisors, during adolescence, drift mesially by ~0.3 mm per year.[23] In the vertical dimension, the maxillary molars (~1.2 mm/y) and incisors (~1 mm/y) erupt slightly more than the mandibular molars (~0.9 mm/y) and incisors (~0.9 mm/y).[23] Therefore, as the jaws are displaced downward and forward during growth, teeth erupt to fill the space and to maintain the functional occlusion. This eruption of teeth contributes greatly to the vertical dentoalveolar growth in the maxilla and mandible.[23] The final position of teeth within the jaws are influenced by the balance established by the pressure from the tongue, lips, and cheek musculature.

## GROWTH MODIFICATION

The dentofacial orthopedic intervention, by an orthodontist, is an attempt to modify growth to correct the developing skeletal discrepancies. In routine orthodontic diagnosis, the discrepancies in growth are analyzed in 3 dimensions: (1) transverse, (2) sagittal, and (3) vertical planes of space. The widespread consensus, albeit there are individual variations, is that transverse growth is completed first, then the sagittal growth, and finally, the vertical growth.

### Transverse Dimension

Skeletal discrepancies in the transverse dimension manifest as (1) constricted or wide maxilla, and/or (2) constricted or wide mandible. The growth modification of constricted maxilla is often achieved with palatal expansion. In children at the age group of 8 or 9 years of age, expansion of the midpalatal suture is easily achieved with little force using tooth-supported appliances, such as W-arch or Quad Helix.[24] However, children who are 10 years or older require heavier forces to open the interdigitated midpalatal suture. Therefore, correction of maxillary constriction at ~10 years of age often requires jackscrew devices to create micro-fractures to open the midpalatal suture.[24] Although the goal of expansion is to produce skeletal changes, it is not always the case. The tooth-supported palatal expansion devices produce approximately 50% dental and 50% skeletal expansion.[24]

The uncorrected maxillary constriction at adolescent age group presents a major challenge in opening the midpalatal suture with tooth-supported jackscrew devices. This is because the heavier forces delivered with such devices often fail to open the suture and will cause dental tipping and in some cases may cause buccal bone fracture. The advent of miniscrews in orthodontic treatment allows delivering forces directly to the midpalatal suture in achieving true sutural split.[25] The miniscrew-assisted rapid palatal expander is a useful modality to correct maxillary constriction in young adults who might otherwise require surgery.

Unlike the maxilla, expansion of the constricted mandible is possible only with surgical approach, such as distraction osteogenesis due to early ossification of the midline mandibular cartilage.[24] Currently, there are no viable growth modification modalities to correct excessive transverse maxillary or mandibular growth, and surgery is the only treatment of choice.

### Sagittal Dimension

In the sagittal dimension, the skeletal discrepancies manifest as (1) Class II skeletal relationship due to prognathic maxilla and/or retrognathic mandible, and (2) Class III skeletal relationship due to retrognathic maxilla and/or prognathic mandible. The 2 major growth modification modalities for Class II growth pattern are (1) traction with extraoral forces, such as head gear; and (2) functional appliances, such as Twin Block, Bionator, and Herbst appliances. In Class II skeletal discrepancy due to excessive maxillary growth, or in some situations with normal maxilla and retrognathic mandible, extraoral traction with head gear is a reasonable treatment modality.[24] The head gear therapy before or during adolescence delivers compressive forces to the circummaxillary sutures in restraining the forward maxillary growth and allows the mandible to catch up to its inherent genetically determined growth potential. The second treatment modality of functional appliance therapy has been surrounded with much controversy in the orthodontic literature. Increasing evidence supports the notion that, on a short-term basis, functional appliance therapy before or during adolescence accelerates forward mandibular growth, but *not* any more than the inherently determined genetic potential. Generally, the functional appliances tend to have some restraining effect on the maxilla, with a significant part of the Class II correction achieved through dentoalveolar rather than skeletal changes.[24,26,27] The current consensus, based on multiple clinical trials, with regard to Class II growth modification is that 2-phase treatment during adolescence is not any more effective than 1-phase treatment during adolescence.[24] Therefore, early treatment is indicated when psycho-social burden is a major concern.

The currently available treatment approaches for growth modification in Class III growth pattern are facemask (Reverse Pull Headgear), chin-cup, and Class III elastics affixed to skeletal anchorage. In patients with deficient maxillary growth, facemask therapy is indicated, and the goal of the intervention is to bring the maxilla forward and downward. During facemask therapy, protraction forces are applied to the maxilla with elastics attached from a fixed intraoral appliance to an extraoral facemask. The facemask therapy is effective before 8 to 10 years of age in producing improved skeletal and dental changes.[24,28] During facemask therapy, in addition to maxillary protraction, it is not uncommon to find backward rotation of mandible.

In the continuum of Class III skeletal discrepancy, excessive mandibular growth is on the other end of the spectrum. In these patients, the goal is to attempt to restrain mandibular growth with chin-cup therapy. This therapy involves a cup or cap on the chin with an attachment to the back of the head. The Class III patients with a short face benefit the most by chin-cup therapy.[24] Although the goal of this therapy is to restrain mandibular growth, it almost always results in reduction of chin projection by redirection of condylar growth; backward rotation of the mandible with minimal or no restraint in the actual length of the mandible. Therefore, chin-cup therapy may actually worsen the profile in individuals with a long-face Class III growth pattern. Chin-cup therapy is effective at an early age; however, the circumpubertal growth of the mandible may reverse the effects of early chin-cup therapy.[28]

The usage of elastics to bone anchor plates is growing in popularity. The miniplates are inserted in the infrazygomatic crest and in the mandibular canine region, and Class III elastics are worn from the maxillary to the mandibular miniplates to correct the Class III skeletal growth. The suitable timing of intervention for this modality is ~11 years or older, as this would allow for stable anchorage in the infrazygomatic crest and avoidance of tooth buds. This therapy appears effective in producing maxillary protraction while minimizing side effects like dentoalveolar changes and backward rotation of the mandible.[24]

### Vertical Dimension

The manifestation of skeletal discrepancies in the vertical dimension are (1) short-face and (2) long-face problems. Often times, these problems may manifest along with skeletal Class II or III growth pattern. In individuals with short-face problems, typically the lower facial third is smaller than the upper and the middle facial thirds. The short-face individuals will present with long ramus, acute gonial angle, and hypodivergent mandibular plane angle.[24] The aim of growth modification in these individuals is to allow for the vertical dentoalveolar changes by eruption of posterior teeth. Appliances such as activator or bionator with palatal acrylic contacting the mandibular incisors and interocclusal clearance in the posterior region would allow eruption of maxillary and mandibular molars. Such vertical dentoalveolar changes could improve the short face height.

Contrary to the short-face phenotype, is individuals with large lower facial third, short ramus,

obtuse gonial angle, and steep mandibular plane angle. The growth modification in long-face individuals is rather challenging and difficult. Theoretically, growth modification in growing long-face individuals could be achieved with high-pull head gear to restrain downward maxillary growth with posterior bite block to impede the eruption of teeth and auto-rotate the mandible in the forward direction.[24] However, such a growth modification approach not always produces the desired skeletal changes predictably in the long-face individuals. Interestingly, miniscrew implants provide a unique opportunity for intervention in adolescents with long face. Available limited data suggest that, in growing hyperdivergent patients, miniscrew implants in the palate and mandible with rigid attachment to intrude the upper and lower posterior teeth could prevent the eruption of teeth, improve chin projection, decrease mandibular plane angle, and improve facial convexity.[29]

## SUMMARY

The development of the craniofacial skeleton occurs as a result of a sequence of normal developmental events: (1) brain growth and development, (2) optic pathway development, (3) speech and swallowing development, (4) airway and pharyngeal development, (5) muscle development, and (6) tooth development and eruption. As an orthodontist or surgeon, it is important to understand the growth and development of each subunit of the face so treatment can either harness and manipulate growth or is timed appropriately so as to minimize negative impact. Orthopedic appliances can often be used during growth phases to attempt to manipulate growth favorably. In contrast, it is often ideal if elective surgical interventions are timed when most growth and development is complete so as to not interfere with growth potential.

## DISCLOSURE

The authors have nothing to disclose.

## REFERENCES

1. Valadian I, Porter D. Physical growth and development: from conception to maturity. Boston: John Wright-PSG; 1977.
2. Moss ML, Salentijn L. The primary role of functional matrices in facial growth. Am J Orthod 1969;55(6): 566–77.
3. Ferguson DJ, McDonald RE, Avery DR. Dentistry for the child and adolescent. 7th edition. Philadelphia: Mosby; 2000.

4. Scott JH. The cartilage of the nasal septum: a contribution to the study of facial growth. Br Dent J 1953;95:37–43.

5. Enlow DH, Hans M. Essentials of facial growth. Philadelphia: Saunders; 1996.

6. Lenton KA, Nacamuli RP, Wan DC, et al. Cranial suture biology. Curr Top Dev Biol 2005;66:287–328.

7. Baume LJ. Principles of cephalofacial development revealed by experimental biology. Am J Orthod 1961;47(12):881–901.

8. Koski K. Cranial growth centers: facts or fallacies? Am J Orthod 1968;54(8):566–83.

9. Enlow DH, Kuroda T, Lewis AB. The morphological and morphogenetic basis for craniofacial form and pattern. Angle Orthod 1971;41(3):161–88.

10. Farkas LG, Posnick JC, Hreczko TM. Anthropometric growth study of the head. Cleft Palate Craniofac J 1992;29(4):303–8.

11. Adamo MA, Pollack IF. Current management of craniosynostosis. Neurosurg Q 2009;19(2):82–7.

12. Waitzman AA, Posnick JC, Armstrong DC, et al. Craniofacial skeletal measurements based on computed tomography: Part I. Accuracy and reproducibility. Cleft Palate Craniofac J 1992;29(2):112–7.

13. Waitzman AA, Posnick JC, Armstrong DC, et al. Craniofacial skeletal measurements based on computed tomography: Part II. Normal values and growth trends. Cleft Palate Craniofac J 1992;29(2):118–28.

14. Funamura JL, Sykes JM. Pediatric septorhinoplasty. Facial Plast Surg Clin North Am 2014;22(4):503–8.

15. Johnson MD. Management of pediatric nasal surgery (rhinoplasty). Facial Plast Surg Clin North Am 2017;25(2):211–21.

16. Behrents RG, Harris EF. The premaxillary-maxillary suture and orthodontic mechanotherapy. Am J Orthod Dentofacial Orthop 1991;99(1):1–6.

17. Melsen B. Palatal growth studied on human autopsy material. A histologic microradiographic study. Am J Orthod 1975;68(1):42–54.

18. Persson M, Thilander B. Palatal suture closure in man from 15 to 35 years of age. Am J Orthod 1977;72(1):42–52.

19. Precious DS, Delaire J, Hoffman CD. The effects of nasomaxillary injury on future facial growth. Oral Surg Oral Med Oral Pathol 1988;66(5):525–30.

20. Costello BJ, Rivera RD, Shand J, et al. Growth and development considerations for craniomaxillofacial surgery. Oral Maxillofac Surg Clin North Am 2012;24(3):377–96.

21. Juuri E, Balic A. The biology underlying abnormalities of tooth number in humans. J Dent Res 2017;96(11):1248–56.

22. Marks SCJ, Schroeder HE. Tooth eruption: theories and facts. Anat Rec 1996;245(2):374–93.

23. Buschang PH, Roldan SI, Tadlock LP. Guidelines for assessing the growth and development of orthodontic patients. Semin Orthod 2017;23(4):321–35.

24. De Clerck HJ, Proffit WR. Growth modification of the face: a current perspective with emphasis on Class III treatment. Am J Orthod Dentofacial Orthop 2015;148(1):37–46.

25. Lee KJ, Choi S-H, Choi T-H, et al. Maxillary transverse expansion in adults: rationale, appliance design, and treatment outcomes. Semin Orthod 2018;24(1):52–65.

26. Vaid NR, Doshi VM, Vandekar MJ. Class II treatment with functional appliances: a meta-analysis of short-term treatment effects. Semin Orthod 2014;20(4):324–38.

27. D'Antò V, Bucci R, Franchi L, et al. Class II functional orthopaedic treatment: a systematic review of systematic reviews. J Oral Rehabil 2015;42(8):624–42.

28. Woon SC, Thiruvenkatachari B. Early orthodontic treatment for Class III malocclusion: a systematic review and meta-analysis. Am J Orthod Dentofacial Orthop 2017;151(1):28–52.

29. Buschang PH, Carrillo R, Rossouw PE. Orthopedic correction of growing hyperdivergent, retrognathic patients with miniscrew implants. J Oral Maxillofac Surg 2011;69(3):754–62.

# An Overview of Timeline of Interventions in the Continuum of Cleft Lip and Palate Care

David Yates, DMD, MD[a], Veerasathpurush Allareddy, BDS, PhD[b],*,
Jennifer Caplin, DMD, MS[b], Sumit Yadav, MDS, PhD[c],
Michael R. Markiewicz, DDS, MPH, MD[d,e,f,g]

## KEYWORDS

- Cleft lip and palate • Timeline of interventions • Orthognathic surgery • Lip repair • Palate repair
- Alveolar bone grafting • Cleft maxilla

## KEY POINTS

- Many health care providers are involved in the continuum of cleft lip and palate care.
- Communication between providers is pivotal to realize good end-of-treatment outcomes.
- Treatment philosophies vary across craniofacial teams.

## BACKGROUND

Cleft lip and/or palate (CL/P) is the most common congenital craniofacial anomaly, with a prevalence of 1 in 700 live births.[1–3] According to the US Centers for Disease Control and Prevention, each year 2650 babies are born with a cleft palate, and 4440 babies are born with a cleft lip with or without a cleft palate in the United States.[2,3] Clefts can be unilateral or bilateral, complete or incomplete and involve the alveolus, lip, and/or palate in various combinations. The highest rates of CL/P are reported in Asian populations (0.8–3.7 cases per 1000 individuals), while the lowest rates are reported in Africans (0.2–1.7 cases per 1000 individuals).[4,5] Both genetic and environmental factors have been associated with the development of CL/P. Some of the environmental factors implicated include maternal smoking and alcohol consumption, poor nutrition, and viral infections.[6] Over 350 genes and 300 syndromes have been associated with CL/P.[7] Genes associated with nonsyndromic CL/P include IRF6, 8q24, WNT3, 10q25, and RFC1.[8–11] In addition to traditional polymorphisms, certain methylation patterns have also been associated with an increase risk in CL/.[12,13] A child born with CL/P is typically followed at a cleft/craniofacial center where many specialists

[a] EPCH Cleft and Craniofacial Fellowship, El Paso Children's Hospital, TTUHSC, El Paso – Paul Foster School of Medicine, High Desert Oral & Facial Surgery, 601 Sunland Park Drive, bldg 2, suite 2, El Paso, TX 79912, USA; [b] Department of Orthodontics, College of Dentistry, University of Illinois at Chicago, 801 South Paulina Street, 138AD (MC841), Chicago, IL 60612-7211, USA; [c] Department of Craniofacial Sciences, University of Connecticut School of Dental Medicine, 263 Farmington Avenue, Farmington, CT 06030, USA; [d] Department of Oral and Maxillofacial Surgery, School of Dental Medicine, University at Buffalo, 3435 Main Street 119 Squire Hall Buffalo, NY 14214, USA; [e] Department of Neurosurgery, Jacobs School of Medicine and Biomedical Sciences, Buffalo, NY, USA; [f] Divison of Pediatric Surgery, Department of Surgery, Jacobs School of Medicine and Biomedical Sciences, Buffalo, NY, USA; [g] Craniofacial Center of Western New York, John Oishei Children's Hospital, Buffalo, NY, USA
* Corresponding author.
E-mail address: sath@uic.edu

Oral Maxillofacial Surg Clin N Am 32 (2020) 177–186
https://doi.org/10.1016/j.coms.2020.01.001

are involved in the continuum of care. The objective of this article is to provide an overview of major dental and surgical interventions that are performed in patients with CL/P.

If not treated appropriately in a timely manner, those with CL/P can experience catastrophic events such as premature death and life-long difficulties in feeding, speaking, hearing, self-esteem, and psychosocial relationships.[14–16] The earliest intervention in those with CL/P starts during the first few weeks of life (infant orthopedic treatment performed by a pediatric dentist or orthodontist in preparation for repair of the lip), and the final phase of treatment is comprehensive orthodontic treatment (with/without orthognathic surgery) that is usually performed in the late teen years. Dentists play a crucial role in the continuum of cleft lip and palate care (**Table 1**); therefore it becomes critical that dentists are knowledgeable of the treatment protocols and timing.[17] An overview of the timeline of interventions for the CL/P patient is presented in **Table 1**.

**Table 1**
**Overview of the timeline of interventions in patients with cleft lip/palate and the providers involved at each stage**

| Chronologic Age | Dental Development | Interventions | Providers |
|---|---|---|---|
| By 6 mo | Predentition | Infant orthopedic treatment | Orthodontist and/or pediatric dentist |
| | | Lip repair | Cleft and craniofacial surgeon |
| 10–24 mo | Primary dentition | Palate repair | Cleft and craniofacial surgeon |
| 1–2 y | Primary dentition | Establishment of dental home (and follow every 6 mo) | Pediatric dentist |
| 2.5–3 y | Primary dentition | Speech assessment and velopharyngeal surgery (if indicated) | Cleft/craniofacial surgeon |
| 5–10 y | Primary dentition and mixed dentition | Assess timing of maxillary (alveolar) bone grafting | Orthodontist/pediatric dentist/ cleft and craniofacial surgeon |
| | | Maxillary expansion to establish arch forms and correct posterior cross-bites | Orthodontist |
| | | Maxillary (alveolar) bone grafting | Cleft and craniofacial surgeon |
| 9–12 y | Early to late mixed dentition | Limited orthodontic treatment following maxillary (alveolar) bone grafting | Orthodontist |
| | | Orthopedic treatment using face mask/reverse pull head gear | Orthodontist |
| 12–14 y | Permanent dentition | Bone plate-supported class 3 elastics to correct maxillary/ mandibular antero-posterior discrepancies | Orthodontist and cleft/ craniofacial surgeon |
| | | Maxillary distraction osteogenesis (if there is large maxillary/mandibular antero-posterior discrepancy) | Orthodontist and cleft/ craniofacial surgeon |
| | | Comprehensive phase of orthodontic treatment (if determined that there will not be a need for orthognathic surgery) | Orthodontist |
| >14 y | Permanent dentition | Comprehensive orthodontic treatment (with or without orthognathic surgery) | Orthodontist |
| | | Orthognathic surgery (following completion of growth) | Cleft/craniofacial surgeon |
| | | Final restorative treatment | Periodontist/prosthodontist/ primary care dentist |

## PRESURGICAL INFANT ORTHOPEDIC TREATMENT

Presurgical infant orthopedic treatment (PSIOT) is often the first major clinical intervention that is performed on patients with CL/P. PSIOT is initiated within the first few weeks of life, before surgical repair of the lip. PSIOT is purported to restore the skeletal, cartilaginous, and soft tissue anatomic relationship prior to lip repair and consequently enhance the surgical outcomes.[18,19] Facial tapes, Latham appliances, and Naso alveolar molding (NAM) technique have been widely used for PSIOT (**Figs. 1**). Nasoalveolar Molding for Unilateral and Bilateral Cleft Lip Repair by Kapadia and colleagues in this issue provide an overview of the NAM approach and Dentofacial Orthopedics for the Cleft Patient: The Latham Approach by Allareddy and colleagues in this issue provide an overview of Latham approach for PSIOT. Certain craniofacial centers elect to perform PSIOT only if there is a large defect, while several others do not perform any type of PSIOT.[20] There has been considerable controversy regarding the long-term efficacy of PSIOT and its and adverse impact on maxillary growth.[21] Studies originating from Europe have shown that PSIOT is not an effective intervention and recommend against it.[22,23] However, several craniofacial centers in the United States elect to perform PSIOT with varying degrees of success. A recent survey suggested that half of craniofacial teams reported offering PSIOT, with the NAM technique being the most popular.[20] Grayson and colleagues[24–26] have demonstrated that use of NAM is associated with improvements in nasal angle and increases of nostril width, columellar height, and columellar width.[27]

## LIP REPAIR

Primary cleft lip repair is the first surgical procedure that is undertaken by the surgical team (**Fig. 2**). The repair is generally performed between the ages of 3 and 6 months with the purpose of establishing lip competence by the unification of the underlying orbicularis oris muscle.[28] Lip competence is essential for feeding, speech, and control of oral secretions. There are multiple different techniques for closure of the unilateral cleft lip defect, with the most popular including the Millard technique, the Fisher unilateral cleft lip technique, and Mohler technique. All techniques share in common the need to increase lip height on the affected side by regional geometric flaps; however, each technique approaches this problem differently.[29] The surgical technique for a bilateral cleft lip repair is generally approached in a more standard fashion across all centers. The need for primary rhinoplasty at the time of lip surgery has been fiercely debated throughout the years. Most surgeons have incorporated at least a minimal nasal dissection at the time of the primary lip surgery, convinced that it leads to better nasal outcomes and does not significantly increase the risk of nasal stenosis.[30] It is essential that prior to taking the child to the operating

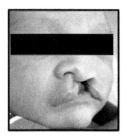 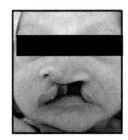 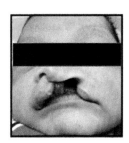 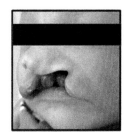

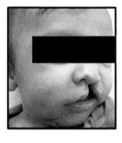 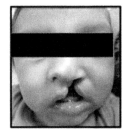 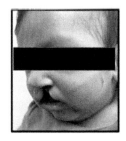

**Fig. 1.** NAM performed by Dr Lizbeth Holguin. Defect size pre-NAM 24 mm; post-NAM 4 mm. (*Courtesy of* Lizbeth Holguin, DDS, El Paso, TX.)

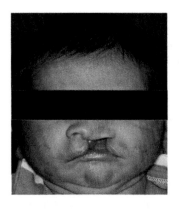 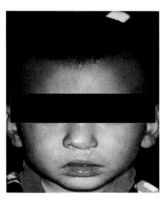

Fig. 2. Preoperative/postoperative lip repair (surgery by Dr David Yates).

room for a cleft lip repair that the patient has undergone an evaluation to assess hearing. Ninety percent of cleft patients will have conductive hearing loss secondary to incompetent drainage of the eustachian tube into the nasopharynx. Tympanostomy tubes are able to relieve this obstruction and may be placed simultaneously with the lip repair, thereby sparing the child an additional anesthesia event.

## PALATE REPAIR

The palate is essential for velopharyngeal competence, which leads to proper speech development and feeding. However, every surgical intervention leads to scarring, and scarring can lead to growth restriction of the nasomaxillary complex. This is why the primary palatal repair is recommended to be performed between the ages 10 to 18 months of age. In this way, one allows unrestricted growth of the palate for as long as possible until speech development demands a repair. There are many different approaches to palatal repair, including: Bardach 2-flap technique, Veau-Wardill-Kilner Pushback technique, von Lagenback bipedicle flap technique, and the Furlow double-opposing Z-Plasty.[31,32] The surgical technique employed should be tailored to each patient, with the goals being to ensure appropriate palatal length, including intravelar veloplasty (repair the levator veli palatini [essential for proper palatal function]), and eliminating anterior palatal fistulae.

## VELOPHARYNGEAL INSUFFICIENCY/ INCOMPETENCE

Velopharyngeal insufficiency/incompetence (VPI) can occur in patients with repaired and unrepaired CL/P. VPI is defined as the ability to completely close the velopharyngeal sphincter that separates the oro- and nasopharynx, which is required for

the normal production of all but the nasal consonants.[33,34] The absence of this ability, termed velopharyngeal insufficiency (VPI), defined as an anatomic or structural defect results from inadequate closure of the velopharyngeal valve.[35] It is seen in a wide range of patients following primary cleft palate repair, with 5% to 40% of cleft palate patients presenting abnormal speech resonance because of residual anatomic structural abnormalities.[36] The primary effects of velopharyngeal insufficiency are nasal air escape and hypernasality. Speech articulation errors (ie, distortions, substitutions, and omissions) are secondary effects of velopharyngeal insufficiency.[34] Children with VPI may have impaired speech intelligibility because of hypernasality, articulation, and low-speech volume. Secondary effects of VPI include nasal regurgitation of liquids, compensatory misarticulations, and facial grimacing. VPI may impact the child's confidence, social development, and overall quality of life.[37]

Velopharyngeal insufficiency can be diagnosed by both subjective and objective means. Along with a thorough medical history, a speech assessment and careful physical examination are required in the children with VPI. The most common diagnostic evaluations of the velopharyngeal function and closure pattern are nasoendoscopy and multiview videofluoroscopy.[38] MRI can be used for examining the anatomy of the velopharyngeal mechanism.[33] Perceptual speech assessment is of central importance in diagnosing VPI and predicting postsurgical outcomes.[37]

Treatment of the VPI falls under the umbrella of 3 main modalities: speech therapy, prosthetic devices, and surgical management. The palatal lifts and palatopharyngeal obturators/pharyngeal bulbs are the most commonly used prosthetic devices. These devices are anchored to the dentition and allow closure of the velopharyngeal port, either by altering the position of the velum (palatal lift prosthesis) or by occupying the pharyngeal gap (pharyngeal bulb).[33] The primary drawbacks to prosthetics are dental caries with concomitant poor dental hygiene, noncompliance, and emotional distress associated with wearing the prosthesis.[39] Noncompliance may be exacerbated by the need for frequent device adjustments, and the number of follow-up visits necessary for proper fitting may be responsible for the further compliance burn.[33] To overcome these drawbacks, a surgical treatment option is available for selected cases. However, the success of the surgical correction of VPI depends as much or more on the selection of the appropriate procedure than on technical expertise.[33] The most commonly used techniques for the surgical management of VPI are furlow palatoplasty, or double-opposing Z-plasty for palatal lengthening; pharyngeal flap; buccinator flaps for palatal lengthening; and dynamic sphincter pharyngoplasty (DSP).

Thorough knowledge of the velopharyngeal anatomy and physiology is critical for understanding the VPI and selecting a specific treatment option to address this condition. Although many different alternatives are available, there is no universal consensus to guide procedure choice, and recent advances in imaging and VPI treatment modalities continue to evolve.

## PREPARATION FOR CLEFT MAXILLARY BONE GRAFTING

Patients with CL/P have collapsed maxillary arches that manifest clinically as posterior and anterior cross-bites (**Fig. 3**). The maxillary arch form is frequently asymmetric, and the minor segment is displaced medially with a collapsed arch adjacent to the cleft. The term alveolar bone grafting is a misnomer, as the entire maxilla is dysmorphic and therefore requires augmentation. A key intervention that an orthodontist or pediatric dentist performs in preparation for the maxillary bone graft procedure is maxillary expansion. Another article provides more details on the techniques of maxillary expansion and associated outcomes. In brief, the indications for maxillary expansion are correction of cross-bites, making maxillary arch compatible with the mandibular arch, and enabling access to the maxillary bone graft site, especially in significantly collapsed arches. Depending on the type and amount of expansion required to achieve the previously mentioned objectives, a wide range of orthodontic appliances (eg, fan-shaped expanders, Haas/Hyrax expanders, and quad helix appliance) may be used.

The timing of maxillary expansion depends to a large extent on the timing of maxillary bone grafting. Thus it is crucial that there is excellent communication among cleft/craniofacial team members, especially between the orthodontist/pediatric dentist and cleft and craniofacial surgeon. It is recommended that maxillary expansion be initiated approximately 6 months before the scheduled maxillary bone graft procedure. The maxillary bone graft procedures must be performed before the eruption of the maxillary permanent canines. The timing of maxillary bone grafts is provided in detail in another article. Typically, the authors evaluate the size and location of the maxillary defect using a combination of periapical, occlusal, and panoramic radiographs. Occasionally, limited field cone beam computed tomography (CBCT) images are also used. If the maxillary defect is present close to the developing permanent central incisor root or permanent lateral incisor root (if this tooth

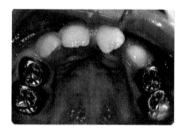
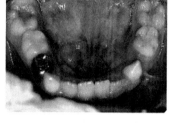
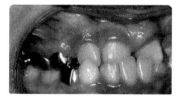
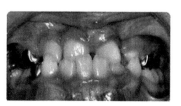
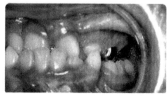

**Fig. 3.** Presentation of a left unilateral complete cleft lip/palate.

is present and viable), then the authors recommend grafting before eruption of the permanent lateral incisor. If there is no viable permanent lateral incisor tooth or if the defect is away from root of a developing permanent central incisor, then the grafting can be done once the root of the permanent canine is approximately 50% to 75% developed and starts to erupt.

## MAXILLARY BONE GRAFTING

Maxillary bone grafting (MBG) is a critical and time-sensitive component of competent cleft care. A successful bone graft provides unity to the maxilla, closes the remaining oral nasal fistula, establishes the nasal skeletal base, and allows the eruption and maintenance of dentition in the area of the cleft.[40] Timing is critical. Bone is unable to be successfully grafted into a defect if any portion of a tooth is in the cleft site. Therefore, it is critical to bone graft prior to tooth eruption into the cleft site. Bone graft timing is dictated by tooth eruption patterns and location of the cleft. If the cleft is more centrally located and the lateral or central incisor could possibly erupt into the cleft, the bone graft should be performed earlier, between 5 and 7 years of age.[41] If the cleft site is more laterally located in the area of the canine, then it may be safe to wait until the patient is between 7 and 11 years of age. Starting at 5 years of age, a cone beam CT is recommended yearly as part of the overall cleft team examination. This radiological examination provides extensive information regarding the size and orientation of the defect, and more importantly, the development of the adjacent teeth.

Expansion prior to grafting needs to be evaluated on a case-by-case basis. In some patients, expansion increases the size of the defect, making the bone graft unlikely to succeed. The other extreme is demonstrated by severe collapse of the maxillary segments, making it impossible to graft because of the inability to access the cleft site. In the first case, it may be wise to graft first and then expand if necessary, whereas in the second example expansion is an absolute requirement prior to grafting. It is critical for the orthodontist, pediatric dentist, and cleft surgeon to all be competent and collaborative in evaluating the dentition and timing of the maxillary bone graft.[42]

Supernumeraries and teeth in the cleft site present a challenge to successful grafting. Patients with cleft lip and palate are prone to supernumerary teeth in and around the cleft site. These are best removed at least 6 weeks prior to the bone graft procedure. By removing these teeth, bone fill is allowed in the extraction sites prior to grafting, making the size of the defect smaller when the actual graft is performed. It also allows time for the mucosa to heal; this will allow the surgeon the maximum amount of tissue possible to work with and manipulate during the actual maxillary bone graft surgery. Malformed or absent laterals are also an issue in the cleft population. Fifty percent of cleft patients do not have lateral incisors on the affected side. Of those patients who do have laterals, 50% are malformed in the cleft population and may need to be extracted prior to the MBG surgery.

Autogenous bone (generally harvested from the iliac crest) is the gold standard for reconstruction of the maxillary cleft site. This has recently been challenged by the use of bone-morphogenetic protein (BMP) mixed with allograft.[43] Both techniques have demonstrated appropriate bone fill and are widely accepted. Additional grafting of the site is often necessary if an implant restoration in the area of the cleft is desired once maxillary growth is complete.

## PREMAXILLARY REPOSITIONING

In the bilateral cleft lip and palate patient it is sometimes necessary to perform premaxillary repositioning surgery at the time of the cleft maxillary bone graft (**Fig. 4**). It is not uncommon for the premaxilla to be so abnormally positioned that a bone graft is actually impossible without its repositioning. Although repositioning of the premaxilla at the time of primary lip surgery is almost always contraindicated and indeed associated with significant maxillary hypoplasia and potential loss, it is sometimes necessary at the bone-grafting stage and can be performed safely and effectively. When performed competently, it will restore the integrity of the maxillary arch, allowing appropriate bone grafting and restoration of the dental arch, aiding in speech and elimination of associated oral nasal fistulae. In the bilateral cleft lip and deformity, it is not uncommon for the premaxilla to be so abnormally positioned that a bone graft is actually impossible without its repositioning.

The blood supply to the premaxilla depends on the nasal septum and the buccal mucosa. The deformity results from the collapse of the lateral alveolar segments and the extension of the premaxilla on the nasal septum. The blood supply to the premaxilla depends on the nasal septum and the buccal mucosa. During the premaxillary setback, a wedge of the nasal septum is removed, and the premaxilla is repositioned and splinted in place.[44] Because of the tenuous blood supply, it is recommended to perform only 1 side of the

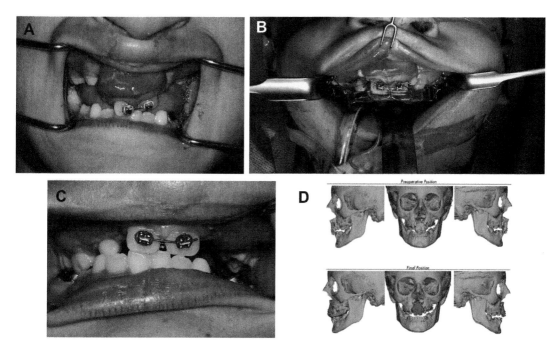

**Fig. 4.** (*A*) Preoperative. (*B*) Premaxillary repositioning. (*C*) Postoperative following premaxillary repositioning. (*D*) Virtual surgical plan and splint placement (surgery by Dr David Yates).

bone graft at the time of the setback and to return to the operating room 8 weeks later to perform a bone graft on the contralateral side. Coordination with the orthodontist is critical to determine the appropriate amount of expansion prior to setback. Virtual surgical planning is helpful in determining the amount of possible and necessary movement. This is ideally performed in the late mixed dentition phase of treatment, and creativity needs to be used in stabilizing and splinting the premaxillary segment after repositioning. Wiring the splint to the dentition with the use of orthodontic wires is preferred but not always possible when securing the splint to the teeth; the use of skeletal anchors to attach the splint is sometimes required.[42]

## LIMITED ORTHODONTIC TREATMENT FOLLOWING MAXILLARY BONE GRAFTING

Frequently, those with CL/P may require a limited phase of orthodontic treatment (usually only in the maxillary arch) following a maxillary bone grafting procedure. This limited phase of orthodontic treatment is performed to facilitate eruption of impacted teeth, correct anterior cross-bites that lead to traumatic occlusion, to align/level the maxillary arch, and to establish compatible arch forms. Occasionally, if the permanent teeth adjacent to a grafted site erupt ectopically, these can be moved into an ideal position with limited orthodontic treatment, and this is by far the most

common indication for limited phase of orthodontic treatment. The movement of the roots of the permanent teeth into the grafted site delivers physiologic stress and thus contributes to the longevity of the grafts.[45–47] It is recommended that radiographs (limited field CBCT or periapical/occlusal radiographs) be exposed to assure the health of the grafted site and maxillary arch continuity before initiating the limited phase of orthodontic treatment. During recent years, bone anchored plates and class 3 elastics have also become popular adjuncts to comprehensive orthodontic treatment, and use of these is thought to minimize the need for orthognathic surgery. This treatment may be initiated during the late mixed dentition stage.

## COMPREHENSIVE PHASE OF ORTHODONTIC TREATMENT

The typical clinical features in patients with CL/P include

Maxillary hypoplasia (this can either be caused by deficient inherent growth potential or restrictions in maxillary growth resulting from scar tissues following the various surgical interventions that occur along the continuum of cleft care)
Class III dental occlusion
Anterior crossbite (negative overjet)

Posterior cross-bite (relative or absolute maxillary/mandibular transverse discrepancy)
Reduced anterior facial height (caused by overclosure)[48–51]

Patients with CL/P almost always require a comprehensive phase of orthodontic treatment that is initiated following eruption of all permanent teeth in the teen years. Depending on the amount of skeletal and occlusal discrepancy, the comprehensive phase of orthodontic treatment is done with or without orthognathic surgery. For those requiring a comprehensive phase of orthodontic treatment in conjunction with orthognathic surgery, it is best to initiate treatment either following cessation of growth or close to completion of growth so as to avoid retreatments. It has been reported that 22% to 40% of patients with CL/P require orthognathic surgery.[48–53] Major drawbacks with large maxillary advancements using classical maxillary osteotomies are high relapse potential and velopharyngeal incompetence and associated speech difficulties.[50,54,55] An alternative to classical maxillary osteotomy for large maxillary advancement is the distraction osteogenesis procedure. The key to long-term success of distraction osteogenesis is retention within the first 6 months following the procedure. Suzuki and colleagues[56] examined a cohort of unilateral cleft lip and palate patients and followed them for 12 months after maxillary distraction osteogenesis and reported dentoskeletal relapse rates of 53.7% in the vertical dimension and 22.3% in the horizontal dimension within the first 6 months. There was no significant relapse during the 6 month to 12 months after surgery. Cho and Kyung[57] followed a cohort of patients with severe cleft maxillary hypoplasia for 6 years after maxillary distraction osteogenesis and reported a 13.5% relapse rate in angular measurements within the first 6 months and only 0.3% relapse from 1 to 6 years.

## RESTORATIVE PHASE

Patients with CL/P frequently having congenitally missing teeth and enamel defects of permanent teeth.[58,59] Maxillary permanent lateral incisors adjacent to the cleft side are frequently congenitally missing or diminutive in size, which often necessitates implants and implant-supported crowns and/or extensive restorative work. The implant phase of treatment is initiated following cessation of skeletal growth. The restorative dentists work closely with the orthodontist to determine the ideal space requirements for placement of implants and implant-supported crowns, and the orthodontist completes the comprehensive phase of treatment, keeping the space requirements in perspective.

## SUMMARY

Patients with CL/P require a multitude of interventions from a myriad of specialists. The earliest intervention is the infant orthopedic treatment of the maxillary alveolus prior to surgical repair of the lip, initiated in the first few months of life. The comprehensive phase of treatment is completed during the late teen years. When a proper team approach to care is taken, excellent outcomes are often realized.

## DISCLOSURE

The authors have nothing to disclose.

## REFERENCES

1. World Health Organization. Global registry and database on craniofacial anomalies. In: Mossey P, Castillia E, editors. WHO reports, human genetics programme: international collaborative research on craniofacial anomalies. Geneva (Switzerland): WHO publications; 2003. p. 15.
2. Parker SE, Mai CT, Canfield MA, et al, for the National Birth Defects Prevention Network. Updated national birth prevalence estimates for selected birth defects in the United States, 2004-2006. Birth Defects Res A Clin Mol Teratol 2010;88:1008–16.
3. Centers for Disease Control and Prevention. Facts about cleft lip and cleft palate. Available at: https://www.cdc.gov/ncbddd/birthdefects/cleftlip.html#ref. Accessed September 1, 2019.
4. Wantia N, Rettinger G. The current understanding of cleft lip malformations. Facial Plast Surg 2002;18(3): 147–53.
5. Vanderas AP. Incidence of cleft lip, cleft palate, and cleft lip and palate among races: a review. Cleft Palate J 1987;24(3):216–25.
6. Mossey PA, Little J, Munger RG, et al. Cleft lip and palate. Lancet 2009;374(9703):1773–85.
7. Funato N, Nakamura M. Identification of shared and unique gene families associated with oral clefts. Int J Oral Sci 2017;9(2):104–9.
8. Imani MM, Mozaffari HR, Sharifi R, et al. Polymorphism of reduced folate carrier 1 (A80G) and non-syndromic cleft lip/palate: a systematic review and meta-analysis. Arch Oral Biol 2019;98:273–9.
9. Li C, Li Z, Zeng X, et al. Is a polymorphism in 10q25 associated with non-syndromic cleft lip with or without cleft palate? A meta-analysis based on limited evidence. Br J Oral Maxillofac Surg 2015;53(1):8–12.
10. Wang B, Gao S, Chen K, et al. Association of the WNT3 polymorphisms and non-syndromic cleft lip

with or without cleft palate: evidence from a meta-analysis. Biosci Rep 2018;38(6). BSR20181676.

11. Wattanawong K, Rattanasiri S, McEvoy M, et al. Association between IRF6 and 8q24 polymorphisms and nonsyndromic cleft lip with or without cleft palate: systematic review and meta-analysis: association of IRF6 and 8Q24 GENES and NSCL/P. Birth Defects Res A Clin Mol Teratol 2016;106(9):773–88.

12. Howe LJ, Richardson TG, Arathimos R, et al. Evidence for DNA methylation mediating genetic liability to non-syndromic cleft lip/palate. Epigenomics 2019;11(2):133–45.

13. Xu XY, Wei XW, Ma W, et al. Genome-wide screening of aberrant methylation loci for nonsyndromic cleft lip. Chin Med J (Engl) 2018;131(17):2055–62.

14. Hunt O, Burden D, Hepper P, et al. The psychosocial effects of cleft lip and palate: a systematic review. Eur J Orthod 2005;27(3):274–85.

15. Hocevar-Boltezar I, Jarc A, Kozelj V. Ear, nose and voice problems in children with orofacial clefts. J Laryngol Otol 2006;120(4):276–81.

16. Geneser M, Allareddy V. Cleft lip and palate. In: Nowak AJ, Christensen J, Mabry TR, et al, editors. Pediatric dentistry - E-book: infancy through adolescence. Philadelphia: Elsevier; 2018. p. 77–87.

17. AAPD Reference Manual. Policy on management of patients with cleft lip/palate and other craniofacial anomalies. American Academy of Pediatric Dentistry 2016. V38, No6, 386-387.

18. McNeil K. Orthodontic procedures in the treatment of congenital cleft palate. Dent Rec (London) 1950; 70:126.

19. Burston WR. The early orthodontic treatment of alveolar clefts. Proc R Soc Med 1965;58:767–72.

20. Khavanin N, Jenny H, Jodeh DS, et al. Cleft and craniofacial team orthodontic care in the United States: a survey of the ACPA. Cleft Palate Craniofac J 2019;56(7):860–6.

21. Berkowitz S, Mejia M, Bystrik A. A comparison of the effects of the Latham-Millard procedure with those of a conservative treatment approach for dental occlusion and facial aesthetics in unilateral and bilateral complete cleft lip and palate: part I. Dental occlusion. Plast Reconstr Surg 2004;113:1–18.

22. Brattström V, Mølsted K, Prahl-Andersen B, et al. The Eurocleft study: intercenter study of treatment outcome in patients with complete cleft lip and palate. Part 2: craniofacial form and nasolabial appearance. Cleft Palate Craniofac J 2005;42(1):69–77.

23. Mølsted K, Brattström V, Prahl-Andersen B, et al. The Eurocleft study: intercenter study of treatment outcome in patients with complete cleft lip and palate. Part 3: dental arch relationships. Cleft Palate Craniofac J 2005;42(1):78–82.

24. Grayson BH, Santiago PE, Brecht LE, et al. Presurgical nasoalveolar molding in infants with cleft lip and palate. Cleft Palate Craniofac J 1999;36(6):486–98.

25. Grayson BH, Cutting CB. Presurgical nasoalveolar orthopedic molding in primary correction of the nose, lip, and alveolus of infants born with unilateral and bilateral clefts. Cleft Palate Craniofac J 2001; 38(3):193–8.

26. Grayson BH, Maull D. Nasoalveolar molding for infants born with clefts of the lip, alveolus, and palate. Clin Plast Surg 2004;31(2):149–58, vii.

27. Nazarian Mobin SS, Karatsonyi A, Vidar EN, et al. Is presurgical nasoalveolar molding therapy more effective in unilateral or bilateral cleft lip-cleft palate patients? Plast Reconstr Surg 2011;127(3):1263–9.

28. Ghali GE, Ringeman JL. Primary bilateral cleft lip/nose repair using a modified millard technique. Atlas Oral Maxillofac Surg Clin North Am 2009;17:117–24.

29. Stals S, Brown RH, Higuera S, et al. Fifty years of the millard rotation-advancement: looking back and moving forward. Plast Reconstr Surg 2009;123(4): 1364–77.

30. Mulliken JB. Bilateral cleft lip. Clin Plast Surg 2004; 31:209–20.

31. Furlow LT Jr. Cleft palate repair by double opposing z-plasty. Plast Reconstr Surg 1986;78(6):724–36.

32. Smith KS, Ugalde CM. Primary palatoplasty using bipedicle flaps (modified von langenbeck technique). Atlas Oral Maxillofac Surg Clin North Am 2009;17:147–56.

33. Gart MS, Gosain AK. Surgical management of velopharyngeal insufficiency. Clin Plast Surg 2014;41(2): 253–70.

34. Fisher DM, Sommerlad BC. Cleft lip, cleft palate, and velopharyngeal insufficiency. Plast Reconstr Surg 2011;128(4):342e–60e.

35. Nam SM. Surgical treatment of velopharyngeal insufficiency. Arch Craniofac Surg 2018;19(3): 163–7.

36. Ahmed M. Cleft lip and palate care in the United Kingdom–the Clinical Standards Advisory Group (CSAG) study. Cleft Palate Craniofac J 2002;39(6):656.

37. Rudnick EF, Sie KC. Velopharyngeal insufficiency: current concepts in diagnosis and management. Curr Opin Otolaryngol Head Neck Surg 2008; 16(6):530–5.

38. Lam DJ, Starr JR, Perkins JA, et al. A comparison of nasendoscopy and multiview videofluoroscopy in assessing velopharyngeal insufficiency. Otolaryngol Head Neck Surg 2006;134(3):394–402.

39. Marsh JL, Wray RC. Speech prosthesis versus pharyngeal flap: a randomized evaluation of the management of velopharyngeal incompetence. Plast Reconstr Surg 1980;65(5):592–4.

40. Precious DS. A new reliable method for alveolar bone grafting at about 6 years of age. J Oral Maxillofac Surg 2009;67:2045–53.

41. Kazemi A, Stearns JW, Fonseca RJ. Secondary graftin in the alveolar cleft patient. Oral Maxillofacial Surg Clin N Am 2002;14:477–90.

42. Rogerson K. Bilateral cleft alveolus surgery. Atlas Oral Maxillofac Surg Clin North Am 1995;3(1):43–9.

43. Dickinson BP, Ashley RK, Wasson KL, et al. Reduced morbidity and improved healing with bone morphogenic protein-2 older patients with alveolar cleft defects. Plast Reconstr Surg 2008; 121(1):209–17.

44. Turvey TA, Ruiz RL, Costello BJ. Surgical correction of midface deficiency in cleft lip and palate malformation. Oral Maxillofacial Surg Clin N Am 2002;14: 491–507.

45. Eppley BL, Sadove AM. Management of alveolar cleft bone grafting—state of art. Cleft Palate Craniofac J 2000;37:229.

46. Guo J, Li C, Zhang Q, et al. Secondary bone grafting for alveolar cleft in children with cleft lip or cleft lip and palate. Cochrane Database Syst Rev 2011;(6): CD008050.

47. Semb G. Alveolar bone grafting. Front Oral Biol 2012;16:124.

48. Ross RB. Treatment variables affecting facial growth in complete unilateral cleft lip and palate. Cleft Palate J 1987;24(1):5–77.

49. DeLuke DM, Marchand A, Robles EC, et al. Facial growth and the need for orthognathic surgery after cleft palate repair: literature review and report of 28 cases. J Oral Maxillofac Surg 1997;55(7):694–7 [discussion: 697–8].

50. Scolozzi P. Distraction osteogenesis in the management of severe maxillary hypoplasia in cleft lip and palate patients. J Craniofac Surg 2008;19(5): 1199–214.

51. Tan SP, Allareddy V, Bruun RA, et al. Effect of infant surgical orthopedic treatment on facial growth in preadolescent children with unilateral and bilateral complete cleft lip and palate. Oral Surg Oral Med Oral Pathol Oral Radiol 2015;120(3):291–8.

52. Rosenstein S, Kernahan D, Dado D, et al. Orthognathic surgery in cleft patients treated by early bone grafting. Plast Reconstr Surg 1991;87(5): 835–92 [discussion: 840–2].

53. Yun-Chia Ku M, Lo LJ, Chen MC, et al. Predicting need for orthognathic surgery in early permanent dentition patients with unilateral cleft lip and palate using receiver operating characteristic analysis. Am J Orthod Dentofacial Orthop 2018;153(3): 405–14.

54. Austin SL, Mattick CR, Waterhouse PJ. Distraction osteogenesis versus orthognathic surgery for the treatment of maxillary hypoplasia in cleft lip and palate patients: a systematic review. Orthod Craniofac Res 2015;18(2):96–108.

55. Cheung LK, Chua HD, Hägg MB. Cleft maxillary distraction versus orthognathic surgery: clinical morbidities and surgical relapse. Plast Reconstr Surg 2006;118(4):996–1008 [discussion: 1009].

56. Suzuki EY, Motohashi N, Ohyama K. Longitudinal dento-skeletal changes in UCLP patients following maxillary distraction osteogenesis using RED system. J Med Dent Sci 2004;51(1):27–33.

57. Cho BC, Kyung HM. Distraction osteogenesis of the hypoplastic midface using a rigid external distraction system: the results of a one- to six-year follow-up. Plast Reconstr Surg 2006;118(5): 1201–12.

58. Jamilian A, Lucchese A, Darnahal A, et al. Cleft sidedness and congenitally missing teeth in patients with cleft lip and palate patients. Prog Orthod 2016; 17:14.

59. Ruiz LA, Maya RR, D'Alpino PH, et al. Prevalence of enamel defects in permanent teeth of patients with complete cleft lip and palate. Cleft Palate Craniofac J 2013;50(4):394–9.

# Dentofacial Orthopedics for the Cleft Patient
## The Latham Approach

Veerasathpurush Allareddy, BDS, PhD[a],[*], Stephen Shusterman, DMD[b],[c], Elizabeth Ross, DDS[d], Victoria Palermo, MD, DDS[e], Pat Ricalde, MD, DDS[f]

KEYWORDS

• Cleft lip • Latham appliance • Lip repair • Infant orthopedic treatment

KEY POINTS

• The primary benefit of presurgical infant dentofacial orthopedic treatment using Latham appliance is that it allows for minimal-dissection gingivoperiosteoplasty.
• In patients with unilateral complete cleft lip and palate, the average reduction in width of cleft using the Latham appliance is 8.7 mm.
• Perioperative complications are minimal.
• Treatment affects long-term skeletal growth of maxilla.

## PRESURGICAL INFANT DENTOFACIAL ORTHOPEDIC TREATMENT

Presurgical infant dentofacial orthopedic treatment (PSIOT) is a process by which cleft maxillary and soft tissue segments can be moved while waiting for surgical reconstruction. Although it can be used in any patient with cleft lip and palate, it is typically reserved for wide cases. McNeil introduced the concept of PSIOT in 1950.[1] Both McNeil and Burston used removable appliances to attempt to stimulate maxillary growth and achieve cleft closure by taking advantage of growth.[1,2] Georgiade and later Latham designed fixed appliances with active mechanics to rotate the palatal segments and, in the case of bilateral complete clefts, to retract the premaxilla to reduce the width of the cleft.[3,4] Millard, a distinguished plastic surgeon known for his work on cleft lip repair techniques, further modified the device and combined it with a surgical protocol that included the gingivoperiosteoplasty.[5] The objective of PSIOT was, and is, to enhance the primary nasolabial repair by repositioning the alar base and restoring the skeletal, cartilaginous, and soft tissue anatomic relationships.[6–8] Repositioning of the maxillary alveolar segments by PSIOT provides a more symmetric maxilla and nasal floor, with a narrower alveolar cleft. In unilateral complete cleft lip and palate, the PSIOT brings together the segments of the maxillary arch in an anatomically neutral position, while neither collapsing nor constricting the maxillary arch form.

## CONTROVERSY SURROUNDING PRESURGICAL INFANT DENTOFACIAL ORTHOPEDIC TREATMENT

The benefit of PSIOT has been widely questioned. The primary benefit is that it allows for

[a] Department of Orthodontics, College of Dentistry, University of Illinois at Chicago, 801 South Paulina Street, 138AD (MC841), Chicago, IL 60612-7211, USA; [b] HarvardSchool of Dental Medicine, 188 Longwood Avenue, Boston, MA 02115, USA; [c] Emeritus, Boston Children's Hospital, 300 Longwood Avenue, Boston, MA 02115, USA; [d] Department of Developmental Biology, Boston Children's Hospital, Harvard School of Dental Medicine, 300 Longwood Avenue, Boston, MA 02115, USA; [e] Florida Craniofacial Institute, 4200 North Armenia Avenue, Tampa, FL 33607, USA; [f] Florida Craniofacial Institute, St. Joseph's Cleft and Craniofacial Center, 4200 North Armenia Avenue, Tampa, FL 33607, USA
* Corresponding author.
E-mail address: sath@uic.edu

Oral Maxillofacial Surg Clin N Am 32 (2020) 187–196
https://doi.org/10.1016/j.coms.2020.01.002
1042-3699/20/© 2020 Elsevier Inc. All rights reserved.

minimal-dissection gingivoperiosteoplasty for teams that have incorporated this procedure into their protocols.[5,7,9] The average change in cleft width reported in a retrospective study of 40 patients with unilateral cleft lip and palate treated with PSIOT with dentomaxillary appliance (DMA) was 8.7 mm (3–13.8 mm).[10] There is considerable controversy regarding the long-term efficacy of PSIOT and its potential adverse impact on maxillary growth. Multicenter studies originating in Europe (Eurocleft and Dutchcleft studies) have suggested that PSIOT is not effective, and there is no uniform consensus on treatment protocols.[11–16] These studies have concluded that the benefits of PSIOT on maxillary arch dimensions are only temporary with no long-term benefit and that the PSIOT is not a cost-effective intervention. Results of Eurocleft studies also call into question whether the added interventions and medical visits needed to accomplish PSIOT may actually decrease outcomes because of lifelong patient and parent fatigue.[11–16] A recent systematic review/meta-analysis showed that PSIOT in patients with nonsyndromic complete cleft lip/palate had no significant effect on multiple treatment outcomes such as feeding and general body growth, facial esthetics, cephalometric measures, maxillary dentoalveolar variables and dental arch relationships, speech and language evaluation, and caregiver-reported outcomes.[17]

Regarding facial growth, a cohort of 54 patients (37 with unilateral and 17 with bilateral complete cleft lip/palate) who had a PSIOT using the Latham protocol was compared with 27 patients (20 unilateral and 7 bilateral complete cleft lip/palate) who did not have PSIOT.[18] Both groups were in early adolescence. The study indicated that patients with unilateral complete cleft lip/palate who underwent PSIOT had a slightly shorter maxillary length (−2.1 mm) and lower anterior facial height (−2.8 mm) compared with those who did not have PSIOT, which suggests that PSIOT with modified Latham appliances results in restriction of maxillary length and lower anterior facial height at that age.

The most powerful longitudinal outcome studies have been reported by Berkowitz and colleagues. Berkowitz looked at patient data spanning 20 years and found those who underwent PSIOT using Latham appliances experienced significant deleterious effects on maxillary growth. This was described as anterior crossbites in unilateral complete cleft lip and palate and buccal crossbites in bilateral complete cleft lip and palate.[19–21] The anteroposterior and vertical dimensions of the maxilla were also shown to be affected.[20,22,23] Berkowitz went on to eloquently describe how the bodily movement of the premaxilla against the premaxillary-vomerine suture created disruption and growth cessation at this very delicate junction, resulting in profound negative consequences. He observed that no further change in the anteroposterior length of the maxilla from first molar to incisor occurred after the premaxilla was retracted in bilateral complete cleft lip and palate patients.[19–21] Ventroflexion of the premaxilla, however, as is seen with taping from cheek to cheek, will only exert slight forces to the premaxilla and does not have the same deleterious effects on growth.

Another concern is dental development and eruption. In a retrospective analysis, the incidence of second premolar agenesis and enamel defects was not seen to be significant between the PSIOT and non-PSIOT groups; however, there was a significant difference regarding ectopic eruption of maxillary molars.[24] In the PSIOT group, ectopic eruption of maxillary molars was seen in 28.4% of patients as compared with 1.4% the non-PSIOT group. Palatal pressure from the acrylic appliances as well as placement of the retention pins could be contributing factors.

Despite the controversies surrounding PSIOT, several craniofacial centers across the United States continue to use this protocol. In this article, the authors present an overview of a PSIOT technique (modified Latham approach), the step-by-step sequence of using this technique, and observations using this protocol.

## OVERVIEW OF LATHAM APPROACH

There are various PSIOT techniques available including nasoalveolar molding, taping systems, bonnets, and the Latham appliance.[25,26] The prime objective of all techniques is to better align the alveolar segments and to narrow the cleft gap before lip repair. Because the major and minor segments are brought in close proximity to each other, the lip segments and the base of the nose are also brought close together. The goal of PSIOT in patients with bilateral complete cleft lip and palate is to widen the palatal segments anteriorly to allow retraction of the premaxilla to a more normal position within the maxillary arch and to minimize tension on the repaired lip. The Latham technique uses an intraoral fixed appliance activated at several intervals.[5,9] If created properly, the Latham appliance can provide precise control over the movements of the major and minor segments of the maxillary arch.

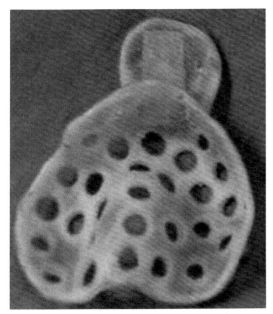

**Fig. 1.** Custom acrylic for obtaining impressions.

## TREATMENT OF UNILATERAL COMPLETE CLEFT LIP AND PALATE WITH THE LATHAM APPROACH

The following is a step-by-step protocol for treatment of patients with unilateral complete cleft lip and palate with the Latham appliance:

- Maxillary arch impression is obtained using a polyvinyl silaxone–based material in a customized impression tray (**Fig. 1**). Setting time can be controlled by varying the amount of accelerator and withholding the material to shorten the intraoral time. The tray must not be overfilled.
- The appliance, referred to as the DMA, is fabricated by a dental laboratory.
- The appliance (**Fig. 2**) is typically composed of an acrylic base connected by a posterior stainless steel hinge and adapted over the major and minor segments of the maxilla, an activating stainless steel screw, and an elastomeric chain.
- The DMA is inserted in the operating room under general anesthesia. The timing of insertion is based on the schedule for lip repair, usually between 3.5 and 5 months of age. The appliance should be in the mouth for no less than 6 weeks.
- The armamentarium used to place the DMA is shown in **Fig. 3**, using standard techniques.
- The appliance is fixed to the maxillary arch by using 4 transmucosal stainless steel pins (0.020 gauge), which are about 15 to 18 mm in total length (**Fig. 4**). The pins are inserted through the acrylic on the medial aspect of each palatal segment at an angle of 30° to 40° from the vertical and placed so as to penetrate the palatal bone while avoiding the developing dentition.
- An appropriately placed DMA is shown in **Fig. 5**.
- The patient remains in the hospital overnight to assure a patent airway, resumption of feeding, and urinary output.
- Following discharge from hospital, the patient is followed at intervals of 1-week, 3-weeks, and 5-weeks.
- Oral or rectal acetaminophen can be given for pain as needed.
- The parent activates the appliance by turning the stainless steel screw one full turn (360°) every day, and the elastomeric chain is activated by the dentist at the 1-week, 3-week, and 5-week follow-up visits.
- Activation continues until the major and minor segments are in close approximation (within

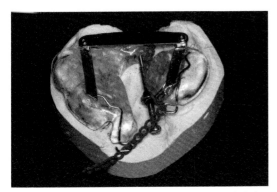

**Fig. 2.** Dentomaxillary appliance for unilateral cleft.

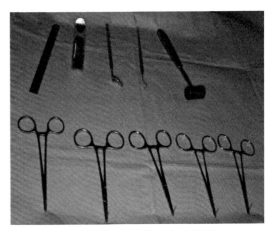

**Fig. 3.** Armamentarium used to place DMA.

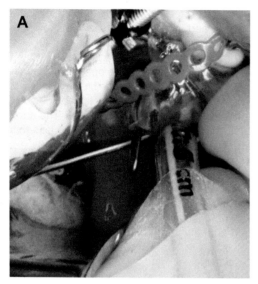
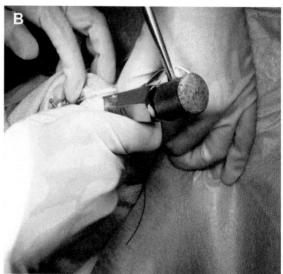
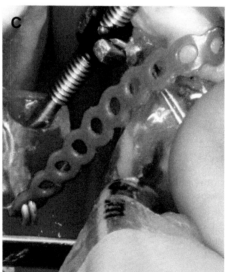

Fig. 4. (A–C) Placement of retaining pins.

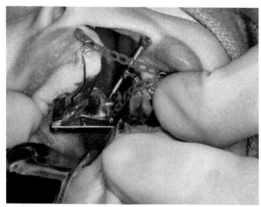

Fig. 5. Well-placed DMA.

1–2 mm) or until it is no longer possible to turn the activating screw.

- Ideal outcome is shown in **Fig. 6**.
- The DMA is removed at the time of lip-nasal repair under the same general anesthetic, and final records may be obtained (**Fig. 7**).

## TREATMENT OF BILATERAL COMPLETE CLEFTS WITH LATHAM APPROACH

The following is a step-by-step sequence of treating patients with bilateral complete cleft lip and palate with a Latham appliance:

- A maxillary arch impression is obtained in a manner similar to the unilateral protocol. It is critical that anatomy of the palatal segments

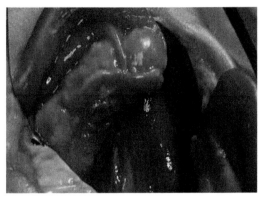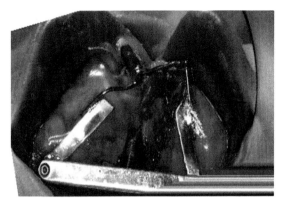

**Fig. 6.** Ideal outcome following PSIOT with DMA in a unilateral cleft.

and the premaxilla are captured in their entirety.

- The appliance used in the treatment of bilateral complete cleft lip and palate is referred to as the elastic chain premaxillary retraction (ECPR) appliance (**Fig. 8**). As in the DMA, the ECPR appliance has acrylic shelves covering the palatal segments, fixed in place with 4 pins. In the case of the ECPR, the

midline posterior hinge includes a ratcheted expansion screw, a trans-premaxillary U-shaped wire threaded through the premaxilla, anterior to the premaxilla-vomer suture, and elastomeric chains to retract the premaxilla.

- The ECPR appliance is inserted under general anesthesia but may be delayed if the bilateral cleft lip is to be repaired later than the

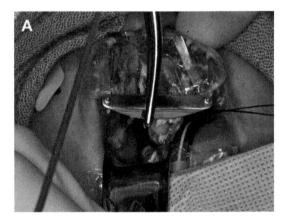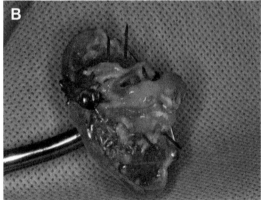

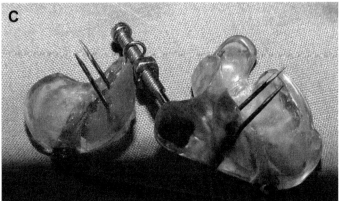

**Fig. 7.** (A–C) Removal of DMA following completion of PSIOT.

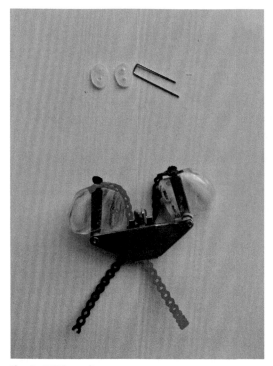

**Fig. 8.** ECPR appliance.

unilateral cleft. It will remain in the mouth for a period of approximately 6 weeks.

- The armamentarium used to place the ECPR is similar to that used for DMA but will include a hand-held chuck and Peeso endodontic burs to drill the dual channels through the premaxillary neck.
- An ECPR is shown in **Fig. 9**.
- The patient remains in the hospital overnight to assure the airway, feeding, and urinary output.
- Following discharge, the patient is followed at 1-week, 3-week, and 5-week intervals.
  - Postoperative medications are similar to those used for unilateral appliance insertion.
- The parent activates the appliance by turning the stainless steel screw one-quarter turn (90°) until an audible or haptic click is heard or perceived every day, and the elastomeric chains are activated by the dentist bilaterally at the 1-week, 3-week, and 5-week follow-up visit intervals. The ECPR appliance is activated until there is sufficient anterior expansion of the palatal segments to accommodate the retracted premaxilla. Care must be exercised to avoid overexpansion of the

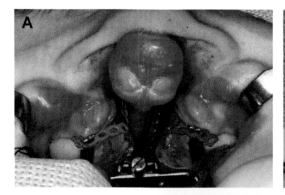
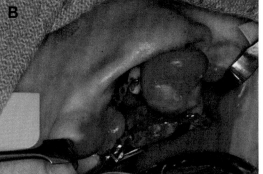
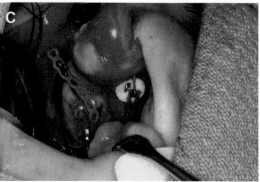

**Fig. 9.** (*A–C*) Ideal ECPR placement.

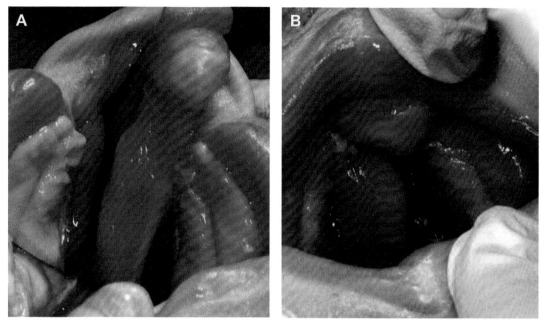

**Fig. 10.** (*A, B*) Pre- and posttreatment ideal outcome following PSIOT with ECPR.

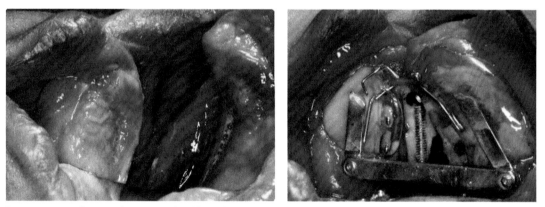

**Fig. 11.** Accumulation of mucus and milk curd, which should be minimized by hygiene efforts.

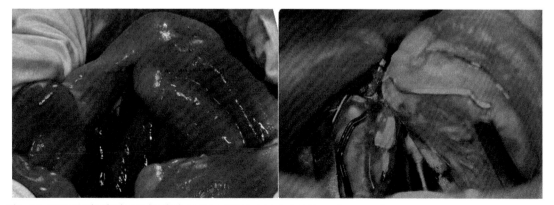

**Fig. 12.** Excessively thick acrylic shelves preventing approximation of segments.

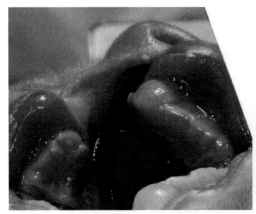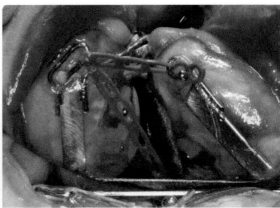

**Fig. 13.** Position of activating screw preventing approximation of segments.

nasal alar cartilages and flattening of the nasal dome.

- An outcome following ECPRPSIOT is shown in **Fig. 10**.
- The ECPR is removed under general anesthesia at the same time as lip-nasal repair.

## PERIOPERATIVE COMPLICATIONS OF THE LATHAM PROTOCOL

Blood loss during the procedure is negligible, with only 5.2% of patients losing greater than 4 mL blood loss.[10] The Latham appliances are bulky intraorally, and some patients have postinsertion feeding difficulty. However, most patients are discharged within 24 hours of insertion. Occasionally the in-hospital stay requires extension to 2 or more nights due to feeding difficulties. Following discharge and after normal feeding has resumed, the most frequently encountered complaint is difficulty maintaining oral hygiene (**Fig. 11**). Mucus and milk curd tend to accumulate on and within the appliance. Despite the appearance and some odor, we do not encourage vigorous cleaning of the appliance. Debris is meticulously removed at the first follow-up visit with suction. Localized inflammation of soft tissues is also common, but recovery is rapid after appliance removal and typically does not delay surgical intervention. Care must be taken during fabrication of the appliances to avoid acrylic interference with palatal segments (**Fig. 12**). The position of the activating screw is also critical. In unilateral complete clefts, the activating screw should be positioned so that it does not interfere with the approximation of the segments nor irritate the soft tissues of the nares (**Fig. 13**). In the authors' experience, appliance or pin retention have not been a problem, but the pins, which are held in place with friction, should be further protected with composite at insertion,

and parents must not be vigorous in cleaning the mouth.

In an attempt to study morbidity, the physiologic and behavioral indicators of pain within the first 24 hours following insertion of either the DMA (n = 82) or the ECPR (n = 27) appliances in a cohort of 109 infants (75 men and 34 women) were observed and recorded.[27] The benchmarks included heart rate, systolic blood pressure, respiratory rate, and The Face, Leg, Activity, Cry, and Consolability (FLACC) pain scale scores. Findings revealed that there was an increase in heart rate immediately following awakening after insertion of the appliance, which returned to baseline levels within 8 hours. The systolic blood pressures also increased postoperatively and remained elevated over the time of evaluation during hospitalization. The respiratory rates were lower than baseline levels following insertion of appliances and remained lower during the evaluation period. Both remained within a safe physiologic range. The FLACC scores increased following insertion of both appliances, peaked at 2 hours postoperatively (between 5–6.3), and then decreased. However, even after 8 hours the FLACC scores remained elevated, with scores around 2.

## SUMMARY

The modified Latham device can be used to effectively and predictably reduce cleft width or to retract the premaxilla before cheilorhinoplasty. Although this technique has been available for over 40 years, how it should be incorporated into cleft treatment team protocols has yet to be elucidated. It is a technique that is controversial. Even though PSIOT has the benefit of allowing for surgeons to incorporate minimally invasive gingivoperiosteoplasty into their treatment protocols, prospective randomized clinical studies are necessary to definitively answer concerns that continue to cloud the inclusion of presurgical treatments in treatment protocols for infants with complete cleft lip and palate.

## DISCLOSURE

The authors have nothing to disclose.

## REFERENCES

1. McNeil K. Orthodontic procedures in the treatment of congenital cleft palate. Dent Rec (London) 1950; 70:126.
2. Burston WR. The early orthodontic treatment of alveolar clefts. Proc R Soc Med 1965;58:767–72.
3. Georgiade NG. The management of premaxillary and maxillary segments in the newborn cleft patient. CleftPalate J 1970;7:411–8.
4. Latham RA. Orthopedic advancement of the cleft maxillary segment: a preliminary report. CleftPalate J 1980;17:227–33.
5. Millard DR Jr, Latham RA. Improved primary surgical and dental treatment of clefts. PlastReconstr Surg 1990;86:856–71.
6. McComb H. Primary correction of unilateral cleft lip nasal deformity: a 10-year review. PlastReconstrSurg 1985;75:791–9.
7. Mulliken JB, Martínez-Pérez D. The principle of rotation advancement for repair of unilateral complete cleft lip and nasal deformity: technical variations and analysis of results. PlastReconstr Surg 1999; 104:1247–60.
8. LaRossa D. The state of the art in cleft palate surgery. CleftPalateCraniofac J 2000;37:225–8.
9. Millard DR, Latham R, Huifen X, et al. Cleft lip and palate treated by presurgical orthopedics, gingivoperiosteoplasty, and lip adhesion (POPLA) compared with previous lip adhesion method: a preliminary study of serial dental casts. PlastReconstr Surg 1999;103(6):1630–44.
10. Allareddy V, Ross E, Bruun R, et al. Operative and immediate postoperative outcomes of using a latham-type dentomaxillary appliance in patients with unilateral complete cleft lip and palate. CleftPalateCraniofac J 2015;52(4):405–10.
11. Bongaarts CA, van 't Hof MA, Prahl-Andersen B, et al. Infant orthopedics has no effect on maxillary arch dimensions in the deciduous dentition of children with complete unilateral cleft lip and palate (Dutchcleft). CleftPalateCraniofac J 2006;43(6): 665–72.
12. Brattström V, Mølsted K, Prahl-Andersen B, et al. The Eurocleft study: intercenter study of treatment outcome in patients with complete cleft lip and palate. Part 2: craniofacial form and nasolabial appearance. CleftPalateCraniofac J 2005;42(1):69–77.
13. Mølsted K, Brattström V, Prahl-Andersen B, et al. The Eurocleft study: intercenter study of treatment outcome in patients with complete cleft lip and palate. Part 3: dental arch relationships. CleftPalateCraniofac J 2005;42(1):78–82.
14. Noverraz RL, Disse MA, Ongkosuwito EM, et al. Transverse dental arch relationship at 9 and 12 years in children with unilateral cleft lip and palate treated with infant orthopedics: a randomized clinical trial (DUTCHCLEFT). ClinOralInvestig 2015; 19(9):2255–65.
15. Prahl C, Kuijpers-Jagtman AM, van't Hof MA, et al. A randomised prospective clinical trial into the effect of infant orthopaedics on maxillary arch dimensions in unilateral cleft lip and palate (Dutchcleft). Eur J Oral Sci 2001;109(5):297–305.
16. Prahl C, Kuijpers-Jagtman AM, Van 't Hof MA, et al. A randomized prospective clinical trial of the effect of infant orthopedics in unilateral cleft lip and palate: prevention of collapse of the alveolar segments (Dutchcleft). CleftPalateCraniofac J 2003;40(4): 337–42.
17. Hosseini HR, Kaklamanos EG, Athanasiou AE. Treatment outcomes of pre-surgical infant orthopedics in patients with non-syndromic cleft lip and/or palate: a systematic review and meta-analysis of randomized controlled trials. PLoS One 2017; 12(7):e0181768.
18. Tan SP, Allareddy V, Bruun RA, et al. Effect of infant surgical orthopedic treatment on facial growth in preadolescent children with unilateral and bilateral complete cleft lip and palate. OralSurgOral Med OralPatholOralRadiol 2015;120(3): 291–8.
19. Berkowitz S, Mejia M, Bystrik A. A comparison of the effects of the Latham-Millard procedure with those of a conservative treatment approach for dental occlusion and facial aesthetics in unilateral and bilateral complete cleft lip and palate: part I. Dental occlusion. PlastReconstr Surg 2004;113:1–18.
20. Berkowitz S. A comparison of treatment results in complete bilateral cleft lip and palate using a conservative approach versus Millard-Latham PSOT procedure. SeminOrthod 1996;2:169–84.
21. Berkowitz S. Letter to the editor. CleftPalateCraniofac J 2016;53(3):377–9.
22. Cho BC. Unilateral complete cleft lip and palate repair using lip adhesion combined with a passive intraoral alveolar molding appliance: surgical results and the effect on the maxillary alveolar arch. PlastReconstr Surg 2006;117:1510–29.
23. Henkel KO, Gundlach KK. Analysis of primary gingivoperiosteoplasty in alveolar cleft repair. Part I: facial growth. J Craniomaxillofac Surg 1997;25:266–9.
24. Lin J, Allareddy V, Ross E, et al. A comparison of mixed dentition dental development in cleft patients

treated with and without the latham-type appliance. PediatrDent 2017;39(1):53–8.

25. Alzain I, Batwa W, Cash A, et al. Presurgical cleft lip and palate orthopedics: an overview. ClinCosmetInvestigDent 2017;9:53–9.

26. Nahai FR, Williams JK, Burstein FD, et al. The management of cleft lip and palate: pathways for treatment and longitudinal assessment. SeminPlast Surg 2005;19(4):275–85.

27. Bronkhorst A, Allareddy V, Allred E, et al. Assessment of morbidity following insertion of fixed preoperative orthopedic appliance in infants with complete cleft lip and palate. OralSurgOral Med OralPatholOralRadiol 2015;119(3):278–84.

# Nasoalveolar Molding for Unilateral and Bilateral Cleft Lip Repair

Hitesh Kapadia, DDS, PhD[a],*, Douglas Olson, DMD, MS[b], Raymond Tse, MD[a], Srinivas M. Susarla, DMD, MD, MPH[a]

## KEYWORDS

- Cleft lip • Cheiloplasty • Nasoalveolar molding • Presurgical infant orthopedics

## KEY POINTS

- Nasoalveolar molding (NAM) is an effective tool for both unilateral and bilateral cleft lip repair.
- In the unilateral cleft lip, NAM appliances act to reduce the gap between the greater and lesser segments and the corresponding lip elements, realign the cleft alar base, elevate the cleft-sided lower lateral cartilage, and straighten the deviated columella.
- In the bilateral cleft lip, NAM functions to reorient the ectopically positioned premaxilla toward the midline and expand the alveolar segments as needed. The nasal form is improved by molding the lower lateral cartilages to achieve symmetry and elongating the columella to increase projection of the nasal tip.

## BACKGROUND

Presurgical infant orthopedics is a collective term to describe a treatment method or appliance designed to lessen the severity of the cleft deformity before primary cheiloplasty and rhinoplasty. The first descriptions of these appliances date back to the seventeenth century. Most of the early appliances sought to retract the protrusive maxilla with an external appliance. With these, there was minimal change to the alveolar segments. Beginning with McNeil's molding plate described in the 1940s to 1950s, there have been several techniques designed to reposition the alveolar segments.[1–5] They range from lip taping to the pin-retained Latham appliance, which retracts the premaxilla and expands the posterior alveolar segments. However, none of these directly affect the primary nasal deformity that characterizes cleft lip and palate. As the most visible manifestation of cleft lip and palate, it can present a significant

surgical challenge and it is common for patients to undergo multiple surgical procedures to improve nasal form. This problem led Grayson and colleagues[6–18] in 1993 to develop an appliance that is able to shape the nasal cartilage while also molding the alveolar process. The technique, termed nasoalveolar molding (NAM), has been shown to improve nasal cartilage symmetry and increase columella length. Since it was originally described, NAM has become a mainstay for the presurgical management of children born with cleft lip and palate.

## GOALS OF NASOALVEOLAR MOLDING

The primary goal of NAM for both unilateral and bilateral clefts is to reduce the severity of the cleft by modifying the position of the alveolar processes and improving the nasal deformity before the primary surgical reconstruction. In unilateral cleft lip and palate (UCLP), the gap between the greater

Funding: There was no funding for this work.
[a] Seattle Children's Hospital, Craniofacial Center, 4800 Sand Point Way Northeast, Seattle, WA 98145, USA;
[b] Craniofacial Center of Western New York, Oishei Children's Outpatient Center, 1001 Main Street, Buffalo, NY 14203, USA
* Corresponding author. Seattle Children's Hospital, Craniofacial Center, 4800 Sand Point Way Northeast, OB. 9.520, Seattle, WA 98145.
E-mail address: hitesh.kapadia@seattlechildrens.org

and lesser alveolar segments is reduced, the lip elements are approximated, the cleft alar base distance is decreased, and the deviated columella is straightened. The collapsed lower lateral alar cartilage on the affected side is elevated and molded to a more symmetric and convex form. For bilateral cleft lip and palate (BCLP), NAM is able to move the ectopic premaxilla toward the midline and into a less protrusive position. The collapsed alveolar segments are expanded, as necessary. The nasal form is changed through increased projection of the nasal tip. The nose is molded to achieve symmetry and the columella is nonsurgically elongated.

## NAM APPLIANCE

The NAM appliance consists of an intraoral acrylic molding plate and intranasal stents. The molding plate allows for approximating the greater and lesser alveolar segments in UCLP; in BCLP, the premaxilla is oriented to the alveolar segments. The nasal stent is made of wire and lined with acrylic. It molds the nasal cartilage on the affected side in UCLP; in BCLP, there are 2 nasal stents, which insert into both nostrils. The retention buttons are acrylic attachments on the anterior aspect of the appliance. They allow placement of orthodontic elastics attached to Steri-Strips (3M Corporation, St Paul, MN), which function to secure the appliance within the mouth. The typical course for NAM treatment entails weekly or biweekly adjustments of the appliance for 3 to 4 months for UCLP and 4 to 6 months for BCLP.

## TREATMENT PLANNING

Because of the variability in presentation of cleft lip and palate, a customized plan is made for each patient before beginning molding. It depends on several factors, including the type and severity of the cleft, age of the infant, and practical considerations. The plan should be developed in conjunction with the surgeon and orthodontist and should involve the cleft team. NAM should ideally begin as soon after birth as possible to exploit the plasticity of the nasal cartilage in early infancy. In addition, the infant is more likely to accept the appliance at an earlier age. There is generally less coordinated hand and finger movement and therefore minimal ability to remove the taping and appliance. Regular follow-up is coordinated with the team to ensure the infant is feeding and gaining weight appropriately before starting molding and while in treatment.

There are occasions when beginning NAM treatment may be delayed or deferred because of a unique presentation of the cleft. For instance, the alveolar segments may be severely collapsed in BCLP, resulting in a blocked-out premaxilla. This condition requires expanding the alveolar segments before molding. If the premaxilla is protrusive, it should be retracted through lip taping before beginning NAM. Another common occurrence is the presence of a neonatal tooth on the cleft margin. These teeth are typically nonviable and have minimal bone support. These teeth should be extracted and the oral soft tissues allowed to heal before beginning molding.

### Lip Taping

Once a decision has been made to move forward with NAM, parents begin lip taping in the time that elapses between initial presentation and beginning NAM. It serves multiple roles: (1) it allows the infant to become accustomed to the use of lip tapes; (2) lip taping can serve as an indicator of how the baby's skin will respond to the adhesive on the skin (there are instances in which the skin is sensitive and alternative tapes or barriers may be considered before starting NAM. This can avoid troubleshooting during active NAM treatment); (3) taping can begin reducing the gap between the alveolar segments in the time it takes to begin NAM.

Lip taping is common to both UCLP and BCLP. A base tape made from a hydrocolloid bandage is applied to the cheeks and maintained for up to 1 week. Steri-Strips are then connected with orthodontic elastic in between them. This tape is then placed from the noncleft side to the cleft side under tension. For BCLP, 2 elastics are used with a Steri-Strip in between and 2 Steri-Strips on either side. The central tape is positioned over the prolabium and the tapes on the outside are stretched onto the cheeks.

### Impression Technique, Appliance Fabrication, and Design

A maxillary and nasal impression is obtained once the infant has been cleared by the medical team to undergo NAM. At minimum, the infant should be healthy and there should be appropriate weight gain. The impression is taken in a clinical setting with the infant awake. In the event there is an airway emergency, there should be a professional who is trained to manage an infant airway.

First, an impression tray is selected based on the size of the maxilla. Heavy-body polysiloxane putty material (Coltène Rapid soft putty, Coltène, Altstätten, Switzerland) is then loaded into the tray. The swaddled infant is held upside down and the impression tray is seated with positive pressure. If the premaxilla is ectopically positioned, it can be moved to the midline just before seating the impression tray. Clear visualization of the airway is possible by gently pushing the dorsal surface of the tongue superiorly with a dental mirror handle. Once the impression material is fully set, the tray is removed and the oral and nasal cavities are confirmed to be free of impression material. The impression should capture the alveolar segments including the premaxilla and the vestibular anatomy, and should extend posteriorly to include the entire alveolus (**Fig. 1**A,C).

At the same time as the palatal impression, an initial record of nasal anatomy may be captured with an impression of the nose. The impression is taken with a light-body siloxane material (Memosil 2 [polyvinylsiloxane], Heraeus Kulzer, Hanau, Germany). During the impression, the eyes are kept closed and the medial canthi captured to serve as a registration for position of the nose (**Fig. 1**B,D).

The impressions are poured in dental stone and the resulting cast is trimmed (**Fig. 1**A,C). Any undercuts are blocked out and the cast coated with a separating agent. The appliance is made from hard, clear, self-cure acrylic that is 2 to 3 mm in thickness. Once set, the frenum attachments are relieved and the walls of the appliance are trimmed to allow 2 mm of space between the appliance and the vestibule. A hole approximately 5 mm in diameter is made, centered in the palatal portion of the appliance, to maintain a patent airway should the appliance become dislodged and block the oral airway. The appliance is now ready for delivery, at which time the retention button will be added.

### Appliance Delivery

Delivery is an important time point, because the appliance is adjusted for the infant and the parents given instructions on its use, taping, and care. The appliance is initially inserted into the mouth and all of the tissues in contact with the acrylic plate are carefully assessed for possible impingement. The most frequently observed sites for possible overextension of the acrylic is in the vestibule or near the midline and/or lateral frena. If this is the

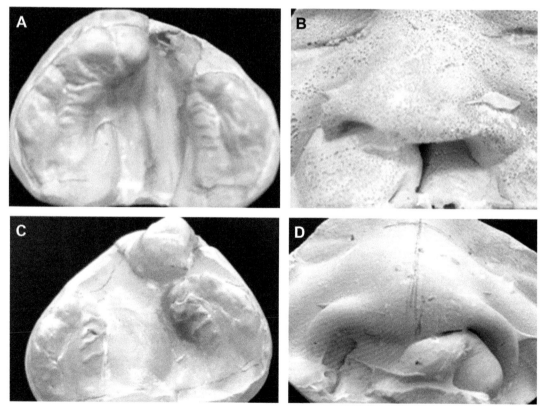

**Fig. 1.** Oral and nasal models for unilateral (*A, B*) and bilateral (*C, D*) cleft lip and palate. The oral impressions should capture the alveolar segments and extend posteriorly to include the entire alveolus. An initial record of the nasal anatomy may be captured with an impression of the nose. The impression is completed with the eyes closed and the medial canthi captured to serve as registration landmarks for the position of the nose.

case, they are marked and the acrylic subsequently relieved.

Once the molding plate is appropriately relieved for a passive fit, the retention button is added to the appliance. For UCLP, the location of the button is between the lip elements, favoring the noncleft side and avoiding impingement of the lip. The rationale for this is that the greater segment moves toward the lesser segment with molding. For a bilateral NAM appliance, the location of the two retention buttons is one on each side of the distal aspect of the premaxilla and between the lip elements. The length of the button is based on the distance required to clear the lips with the retention tapes once attached. To maximize retention of the appliance, the button is added at a 30° to 40° angle to the occlusal plane to allow a slight vertical vector of force to be applied from the tapes.

Retention tapes are fabricated from 6 × 100-mm (0.25 × 4 inch) Steri-Strips and orthodontic elastics (6 mm [0.25 inch] or 5 mm [0.19 inch], 128 g [4.5 oz]). They are used from the acrylic plate and adhere to the cheeks, simultaneously securing the appliance as well as delivering the active force needed for correction. For a UCLP, 2 retention tapes are applied from the single retention button, extending to the left and right cheeks. For a BCLP, 1 retention tape is used from each retention button, extending to the left and right cheeks.

In order to minimize irritation to the cheeks, a base tape made from a hydrocolloid bandage is first applied to each. They are to be placed just outside of the nasolabial creases and below the eyes, at an angle, with the medial portion lower than the lateral portion. The retention tapes, which are frequently changed through the course of a day, are then directly adhered to them. The base tapes can be maintained for up to a week.

### Nasal Molding

The primary objectives of nasal molding include (1) to increase projection of the nasal tip; (2) to obtain symmetry of the lower lateral alar cartilages; (3) nonsurgical lengthening of the columella. Nasal

molding is accomplished through use of a single nasal stent in UCLP and bilateral nasal stents in BCLP (**Fig. 2**). The nasal stents are added to the appliance once the gap between the alveolar segments is 5 mm or less. This reduction in the distance between the alveolar segments allows for elevation of the cleft alar rim when they are under less tension.

The nasal stent consists of 0.91-mm (0.036-inch) round stainless steel wire; hard, clear, self-cure acrylic; and soft denture liner. The wire is embedded into the appliance using acrylic and is bent to give it an accentuated curve allowing for future activations during routine adjustment appointments. The terminal nasal portion is made up of 2 lobes, a superior and inferior, formed from acrylic and covered with soft denture liner. The superior lobe is positioned within the nostril to project the nasal dome and tip. The inferior lobe supports the nostril apex. The nasal stent is gradually adjusted to lift, provide support, and mold the cleft nostrils.

Unique to a BCLP is the use of the nasal stents to provide nonsurgical elongation of the columella. In order to accomplish this, the nasal stents are connected with a band of soft denture liner. This resulting columella band is positioned at the nasolabial junction inferiorly and can gradually be increased in size to elongate the columella. To facilitate this elongation, an additional Steri-Strip with 2 orthodontic elastics can be fabricated and applied from the prolabium to the retention buttons.

## NASOALVEOLAR MOLDING FOR UNILATERAL CLEFT LIP AND PALATE

The goal in molding of the greater and lesser segments in a UCLP is to reduce the space between the 2 segments to 5 mm or less (**Fig. 3**). Decreasing the width between the greater and lesser alveolar segments facilitates reduction in the width of the alar base, thereby minimizing the tension in these tissues.

Reduction of the width between the 2 segments is possible through successive removal of acrylic

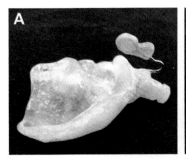
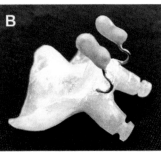

Fig. 2. NAM devices with nasal molding extensions for unilateral (*A*) and bilateral (*B*) cleft lip and palate.

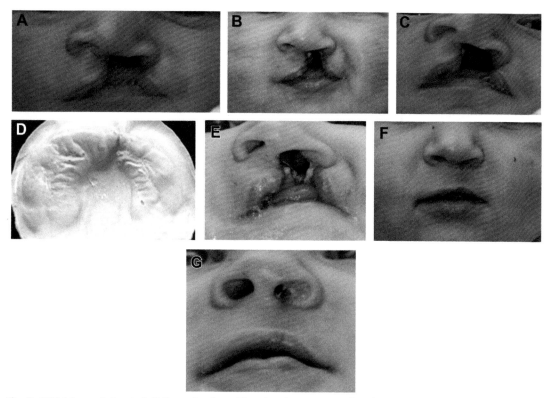

**Fig. 3.** NAM for unilateral cleft lip and palate. The alveolar gap noted in the initial impression (see **Fig. 1**A) is narrowed significantly following NAM (*A*). The apposition of the alveolar segments, molding of the lower lateral cartilage, and narrowing of the alar base results in less tension on the tissues and facilitates surgical repair (*B–G*).

within the molding plate along the lesser segment as selective force is applied through the retention tapes. To avoid impingement of posterior tissues as the appliance rotates, acrylic is removed from the posterior aspect. Throughout the process, the addition of soft denture liner can help detail the correction within the greater and lesser segments. However, care must be taken to maintain equal removal of acrylic and addition of soft denture liner to prevent compression of the alveolar process.

The stepwise removal of acrylic with or without addition of soft denture liner requires weekly or biweekly modification of the appliance. Each adjustment of the appliance is limited to 1 to 2 mm of addition and/or removal of material, which minimizes the potential for developing any pressure sores or irritations. In addition, the appliance tends to be better adapted and more stable with gradual adjustments increasing the infant's tolerance of the treatment. Clinical progress is assessed frequently during the molding process, in anticipation of lip and nasal repair at approximately 6 months of age (**Fig. 3**C–G).

## NASOALVEOLAR MOLDING FOR BILATERAL CLEFT LIP AND PALATE

Alveolar molding in a BCLP is geared toward positioning the often protrusive and ectopic premaxilla between the alveolar segments (**Fig. 4**). This process requires the premaxilla first to be centered to the midline before retraction. Similar to the techniques used with a UCLP, this is accomplished through sequential removal of acrylic and addition of soft denture liner while applying a selective force with the retention tapes. In situations in which the alveolar segments are collapsed palatally, they can and must be expanded through successive removal of acrylic and addition of denture liner before retraction of the premaxilla.

As with a UCLP, care must be taken to remove acrylic from the posterior aspect of the appliance during retraction to avoid impingement of posterior tissues. Gradual removal and/or addition of material is critical to minimize development of sores and maintain a well-fitting appliance throughout treatment. Clinical progress is assessed during the molding process, with changes noted in the premaxillary position, lateral

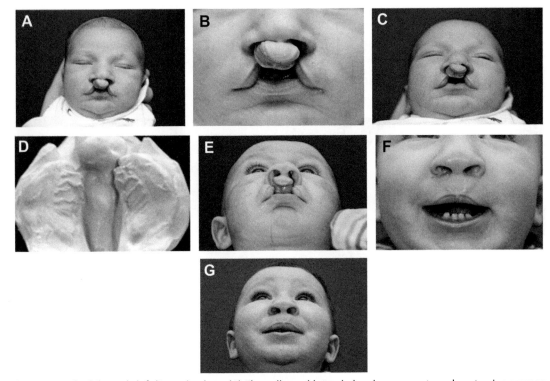

**Fig. 4.** NAM for bilateral cleft lip and palate. (*A*) The collapsed lateral alveolar segments and protrusive premaxilla noted at initial presentation (see **Fig. 1**C) are corrected following NAM (*B*). In addition to these changes, molding of the lower lateral cartilages and nonsurgical lengthening of the columella helps improve results in synchronous lip-nasal repair (*B–G*). The clinical examples/figures are the result of careful planning, coordination, and treatment by the primary orthodontist and senior surgeon (H.K. and R.T.)

alveolar segments, as well as alar base morphology and columella. Synchronous lip and nasal repair is performed at approximately 6 months of age (see **Fig. 4**C–G).

## QUESTIONS FOR CONSIDERATION
### What Is the Impact of Nasoalveolar Molding on Maxillary Growth?

A recent randomized controlled clinical trial evaluating the early effects of NAM on maxillary growth in UCLP showed that NAM is effective for realigning the greater and lesser segments without immediate adverse effects on vertical or transverse arch growth.[1] These findings are consistent with those reported by Fuchigami and colleagues,[11] who, based on a three-dimensional evaluation of dental casts in patients with UCLP, showed that NAM improved maxillary arch morphology and symmetry, as well as nasolabial contour, including columellar positioning.[2] NAM was reported to prevent alveolar width widening with growth.[3] Long-term effects on maxillary growth remain an area of active investigation; such effects may be confounded by surgical technique for lip and palate repair.

### What Are the Outcomes of Nasoalveolar Molding?

Outcomes of NAM have been the subject of several recent investigations. Although generalizations about the effectiveness are limited by heterogeneity between studies, as well as inconsistent follow-up times, a few trends have been observed. A survey study of surgeons evaluating patients with cleft lip plus or minus palate suggests that surgeons assessed the likelihood of revision to be less in patients who underwent NAM.[1] Broder and colleagues[14] report better caregiver-reported outcomes following surgery in patients undergoing NAM versus those who had not undergone NAM.[2] The difference was most notable with regard to nasal appearance. The observation regarding nasal appearance is consistent with data from Barillas and colleagues,[15] who evaluated nasal morphology in patients with nonsyndromic UCLP. These investigators retrospectively assessed 4 nasal anthropometric distances and

2 angular relationships in patients with UCLP who underwent NAM compared with patients with UCLP who underwent surgical correction alone. They report a greater degree of nasal symmetry in patients undergoing NAM at an average of 9 years postoperatively.[3] The same group reported improvements in columellar length and a decreased need for nasal surgery at 3 years of age in patients with BCLP who underwent NAM, compared with those who did not undergo NAM.[4] Subsequent work by this group showed nearly normal nasal morphology at 12.5 years of age in patients with BCLP who were treated with NAM and primary nasal reconstruction at the time of lip repair.[5] As with surgical techniques for management of cleft lip and palate, there are identifiable differences in outcomes for NAM in UCLP versus BCLP.[6] Nostril breadth was more favorably modified in UCLP, as was bialar width. In BCLP, NAM more effectively increases columellar height and width.

### What Are the Risks of Nasoalveolar Molding?

These purported benefits should be weighed against the risks of NAM. A review of NAM-related complications noted that nearly three-quarters of patients had an adverse event related to soft tissue, most commonly ulcerations.[1] Noncompliance was reported to occur 40% of the time. Although these data do not suggest that NAM is a high-risk undertaking, they do stress the importance of team-based, multidisciplinary care for patients with cleft-related differences.

### SUMMARY

NAM is a powerful presurgical technique used to reduce the severity of the cleft through improved alignment of the alveolar segments and lip elements. However, its ability to improve on the primary cleft nasal deformity before surgical correction is unique. This improvement includes increased nasal tip projection, improved symmetry of the lower alar cartilage, and nonsurgical elongation of the columella. Since its introduction, the singular benefits it offers have been recognized by numerous practitioners, leading to its adoption as the treatment of choice at cleft centers throughout the United States, as well as the rest of the world. However, as with choosing any treatment modality regarding UCLP and BCLP, careful consideration needs to be taken regarding the individuality of every case, with decisions ultimately being made following conscientious discussions between the orthodontist, surgeon, cleft team, and patient.

### DISCLOSURE

The authors have nothing to disclose.

### REFERENCES

1. McNeil CK. Congenital cleft palate; a case of congenital cleft palate which required the fitting of a special appliance. Br Dent J 1948;84(7):137–41.
2. McNeil CK. Orthodontic procedures in the treatment of congenital cleft palate. Dent Rec (London) 1950; 70(5):126–32. PubMed PMID: 24537837.
3. Winters JC, Hurwitz DJ. Presurgical orthopedics in the surgical management of unilateral cleft lip and palate. Plast Reconstr Surg 1995;95(4):755–64.
4. Georgiade NG, Latham RA. Maxillary arch alignment in the bilateral cleft lip and palate infant, using pinned coaxial screw appliance. Plast Reconstr Surg 1975;56(1):52–60.
5. Latham RA, Kusy RP, Georgiade NG. An extraorally activated expansion appliance for cleft palate infants. Cleft Palate J 1976;13:253–61.
6. Grayson BH, Garfinkle JS. Early cleft management: the case for nasoalveolar molding. Am J Orthod Dentofacial Orthop 2014;145(2):134–42.
7. Grayson BH, Cutting C, Wood R. Preoperative columella lengthening in bilateral cleft lip and palate. Plast Reconstr Surg 1993;92(7):1422–3.
8. Grayson BH, Santiago PE, Brecht LE, et al. Presurgical nasoalveolar molding in infants with cleft lip and palate. Cleft Palate Craniofac J 1999;36(6):486–98.
9. Grayson BH, Cutting CB. Presurgical nasoalveolar orthopedic molding in primary correction of the nose, lip, and alveolus of infants born with unilateral and bilateral clefts. Cleft Palate Craniofac J 2001; 38(3):193–8.
10. Saad MS, Fata M, Farouk A, et al. Early progressive maxillary changes with nasoalveolar molding: randomized controlled clinical trial. JDR Clin Trans Res 2019. [Epub ahead of print].
11. Fuchigami T, Kimura N, Kibe T, et al. Effects of presurgical nasoalveolar moulding on maxillary arch and nasal form in unilateral cleft lip and palate before lip surgery. Orthod Craniofac Res 2017; 20(4):209–15.
12. Nazarian Mobin SS, Karatsonyi A, Vidar EN, et al. Is presurgical nasoalveolar molding therapy more effective in unilateral or bilateral cleft lip-cleft palate patients? Plast Reconstr Surg 2011;127(3): 1263–9.
13. Rubin MS, Clouston S, Ahmed MM, et al. Assessment of presurgical clefts and predicted surgical outcome in patients treated with and without nasoalveolar molding. J Craniofac Surg 2015;26(1):71–5.
14. Broder HL, Flores RL, Clouston S, et al. Surgeon's and Caregivers' appraisals of primary cleft lip treatment with and without nasoalveolar molding: a

prospective multicenter pilot study. Plast Reconstr Surg 2016;137(3):938–45.

15. Barillas I, Dec W, Warren SM, et al. Nasoalveolar molding improves long-term nasal symmetry in complete unilateral cleft lip-cleft palate patients. Plast Reconstr Surg 2009;123(3):1002–6.

16. Lee CT, Garfinkle JS, Warren SM, et al. Nasoalveolar molding improves appearance of children with bilateral cleft lip-cleft palate. Plast Reconstr Surg 2008; 122(4):1131–7.

17. Garfinkle JS, King TW, Grayson BH, et al. A 12-year anthropometric evaluation of the nose in bilateral cleft lip-cleft palate patients following nasoalveolar molding and cutting bilateral cleft lip and nose reconstruction. Plast Reconstr Surg 2011;127(4): 1659–67.

18. Levy-Bercowski D, Abreu A, DeLeon E, et al. Complications and solutions in presurgical nasoalveolar molding therapy. Cleft Palate Craniofac J 2009; 46(5):521–8.

# Orthodontic Preparation for Secondary Alveolar Bone Grafting in Patients with Complete Cleft Lip and Palate

Veerasathpurush Allareddy, BDS, PhD[a,*], Richard Bruun, DDS[b],
James MacLaine, BDS[c], Michael R. Markiewicz, DDS, MPH, MD[d,e,f,g],
Ramon Ruiz, DMD, MD[h], Mark A. Miller, MD, DMD[i,j,k]

## KEYWORDS

- Cleft lip and palate • Alveolar bone grafting • Maxillary expansion • Differential maxillary expansion

## KEY POINTS

- Cone beam computed tomography (CBCT) can be used effectively to determine the timing of alveolar bone grafting.
- Differential maxillary expansion is frequently required before alveolar bone grafting due to the collapsed maxillary arches manifesting as cross-bites in the anterior and posterior segments.
- Good arch form and predictable outcomes may be realized when differential expansion is well planned.
- Relapse is most common sequelae following maxillary expansion. A fixed transpalatal arch with mesial extension arms (up to canines) is needed to retain expansion.

## BACKGROUND

Children born with a complete cleft lip and palate undergo surgical interventions to repair the lip and palate prior to undergoing alveolar bone grafting. There is considerable debate on timing of lip and palate repairs, which depends largely on the protocols unique to the operating surgeon and/or craniofacial team/center. Typically cleft lip repair is done between 3 and 6 months of age, and palate repair is done between 12 and 24 months. These surgical interventions have been shown to restrict maxillary growth.[1–4] The absence of midpalatal bone and scar tissue traction associated with lip and palate repair are thought to constrict the maxilla in all dimensions. In the mixed dentition stage of dental development those with cleft lip

[a] Department of Orthodontics, College of Dentistry, University of Illinois at Chicago, 801 South Paulina Street, 138AD (MC841), Chicago, IL 60612-7211, USA; [b] Boston Children's Hospital Cleft Lip/Palate and Craniofacial Teams, Department of Dentistry, Harvard School of Dental Medicine, Boston Children's Hospital, 300 Longwood Avenue, Boston, MA 02115, USA; [c] Department of Developmental Biology, Boston Children's Hospital, Harvard School of Dental Medicine, 300 Longwood Avenue, Boston, MA 02115, USA; [d] Department of Oral and Maxillofacial Surgery, School of Dental Medicine, University at Buffalo, 3435 Main Street, 119 Squire Hall, Buffalo, NY 14214, USA; [e] Department of Neurosurgery, Jacobs School of Medicine and Biomedical Sciences, Buffalo, NY, USA; [f] Divison of Pediatric Surgery, Department of Surgery, Jacobs School of Medicine and Biomedical Sciences, Buffalo, NY, USA; [g] Craniofacial Center of Western New York, John Oishei Children's Hospital, Buffalo, NY, USA; [h] Arnold Palmer Hospital For Children, 207 West Gore Street, 3rd Floor, Suite 302, MP 197, Orlando, FL 32806, USA; [i] Department of Oral & Maxillofacial Surgery, UT Health San Antonio, 8210 Floyd Curl Drive, Mail Code 8124, San Antonio, TX 78229-3923, USA; [j] Department of Neurosurgery, UT Health San Antonio, 8210 Floyd Curl Drive, Mail Code 8124, San Antonio, TX 78229-3923, USA; [k] Department of Pediatrics, UT Health San Antonio, 8210 Floyd Curl Drive, Mail Code 8124, San Antonio, TX 78229-3923, USA
* Corresponding author.
*E-mail address:* sath@uic.edu

Oral Maxillofacial Surg Clin N Am 32 (2020) 205–217
https://doi.org/10.1016/j.coms.2020.01.003

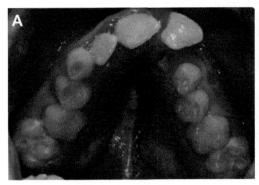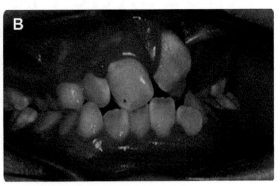

Fig. 1. (*A, B*) Typical occlusal features in a patient with unilateral complete cleft lip and palate.

and palate usually present with anterior cross-bite (negative overjet), a collapsed maxillary arch (predominating in the canine/lateral incisor areas), posterior cross-bite, reduced maxillary arch length, and class 3 occlusion. The typical dentoalveolar features of those with a complete cleft lip and palate are shown in **Fig. 1**. The objective of this article is to provide an overview of the orthodontic preparation prior to secondary alveolar bone grafting of alveolar defects in those with complete cleft lip and palate. The rationale for maxillary expansion, key steps in differential maxillary expansion, and outcomes associated with maxillary expansion are provided in this overview.

## TIMING OF ALVEOLAR BONE GRAFTING

Alveolar grafts should be placed at a time when the bone will be utilized sometime during the following 6 to 18 months. The new bone could be used by a tooth erupting through the area or by an adjacent tooth being orthodontically moved into it. Failure to "load" the bone in the graft area in a reasonable time frame will predispose it to thinning labiolingually and shortening vertically. The exact time

and the amount of load or stress required is truly unknown and an area for research. Practically speaking, however, the orthodontist and surgeon should determine if there is 1 or more useful incisors (good cleft side lateral with enough space to eventually accommodate it) to require a graft in the early mixed dentition. If not, as often is the case with missing or hypoplastic cleft side laterals, the graft is timed based on anticipated eruption of the canine into the graft site. Specifically, the ideal situation is to place a graft knowing that the canine will erupt into the site within a year. This is often estimated by the canine root being two-thirds developed but may also be judged by the cusp tips' proximity to the alveolar plane. So many variations exist that it is impossible to name them all, but commonly the cleft-sided canine is ectopic enough that its eruption path may not be through the graft site. This being the case and if no other tooth is erupting toward the defect timing, of the graft becomes a matter of choice.[5] Occasionally, timing may already be late when the patient is seen, resulting in a situation when a graft must be placed almost immediately. Such a case is demonstrated in **Fig. 2**.

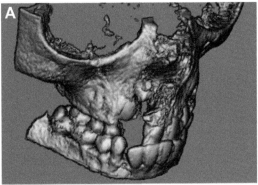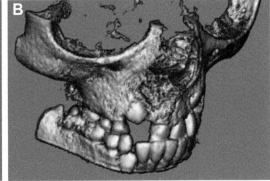

Fig. 2. (*A*) Patient presents with cleft side canine encroaching on alveolar defect. (*B*) Patient 6 months after graft performed 3 weeks after presentation.

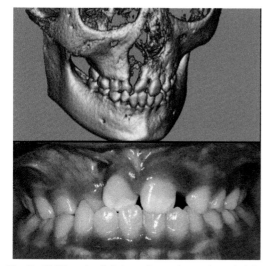

**Fig. 3.** CBCT study of right unilateral complete cleft lip and palate patient whose dentition is pictured.

## EVALUATION OF THE ALVEOLAR DEFECT, NEARBY TEETH, AND OTHER STRUCTURES

Practitioners who have worked in the field long enough will remember the difficulties commonly encountered before the advent of readily available 3-dimensional imaging. The inability to diagnose the defect accurately must have occasionally led to grafts being placed unnecessarily or not being placed when actually needed. Commonly, one could not be sure if a cleft-adjacent tooth could be useful, because its position, size and shape were uncertain. In particular, cleft-adjacent incisors must have adequate bony root coverage in order to optimize graft success. This was often left to the surgeon to determine intraoperatively, a difficult task for certain.

The informed and skilled use of a cone beam computed tomography (CBCT) study solves most all of these problems. In their 2015 overview of cleft orthodontia, Vig and Mercado concluded that CBCTs are "especially valuable" in evaluating cleft lip and palate patients.[6] Step-by-step instructions follow:

1. Obtain a CBCT or CT study of adequate resolution (**Fig. 3**).
2. The surgeon should view it in a program with which he or she has become familiar.
3. Orient the study, if full face or head, in natural head orientation (**Figs. 4** and **5**).
4. Construct 2-dimensional images such as a PAN, lateral ceph, and frontal ceph (**Figs. 6–8**). The surgeon will have the option of temporarily reorienting the study to focus in on a portion of the study and creating additional 2-dimensional images.
5. Evaluate the cleft side canine(s) for root development, orientation, and proximity relative to the bony defect. See **Fig. 9**.
6. Estimate the expected time until eruption into the defect of the above canine(s).

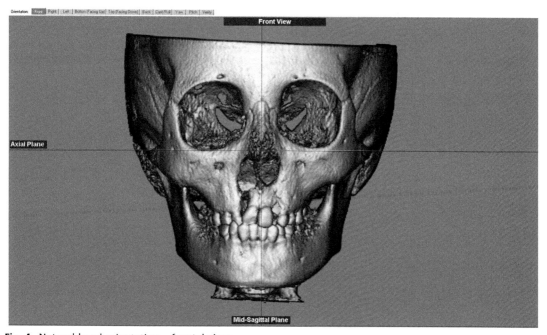

**Fig. 4.** Natural head orientation – frontal view.

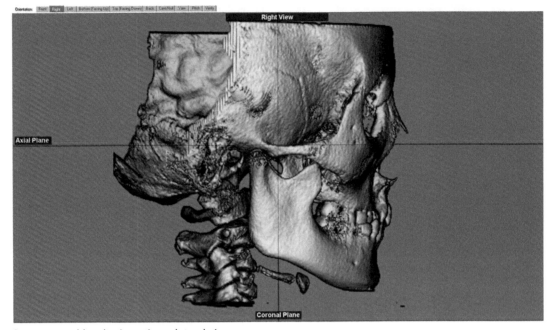

**Fig. 5.** Natural head orientation – lateral view.

7. Orient the study along the long axis of the cleft adjacent incisor and any other tooth of interest.
   a. The study must be viewed in 2 planes, with each oriented along the long axis of the tooth
   b. In the software that the authors use, each orientation may be named and saved (**Figs. 10** and **11**).
8. View each relevant tooth in axial, coronal, and sagittal views to assess bony root coverage. Slice thickness and position along the root must be varied to examine the entire root (**Figs. 12–15**).

9. Make a determination regarding the viability of the above teeth based on the presence of adequate alveolar bone.
10. Use axial slices through alveolar bone to aid in understanding the orientation of the segments. **Fig. 16** shows the anteriorly collapsed minor segment, an orientation that confirms what is seen clinically in the accompanying photograph.
11. For bilateral complete CLP, examine the position of the premaxilla and determine if a premaxillary osteotomy is required.
12. Examine any other teeth of interest (eg, measure the crown size of a supernumerary incisor

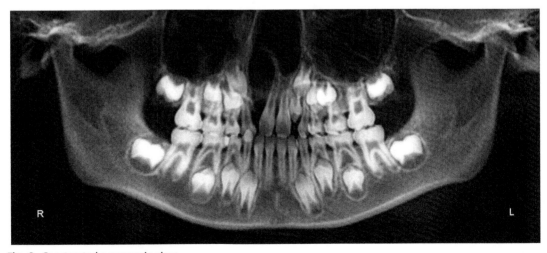

**Fig. 6.** Constructed panoramic view.

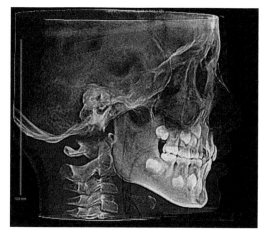

**Fig. 7.** Constructed lateral view.

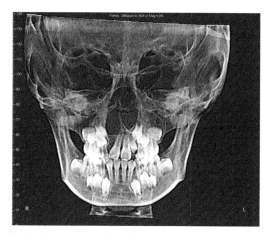

**Fig. 8.** Constructed frontal view.

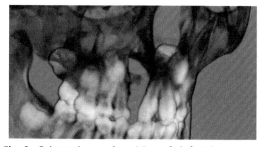

**Fig. 9.** Orientation and position of cleft side canine.

to help determine its future usefulness as seen in **Fig. 17**, and Look at the position of ectopically developing premolars, a common occurrence).

13. The surgeon should share his or her findings and recommendations with the oral and maxillofacial surgeon who will be doing the bone graft. This process is a collaborative one.

The value of a 3-dimensional study, when evaluated carefully, is high and in the authors' opinion worth the x-ray exposure required.

## ORTHODONTIC PREPARATION FOR ALVEOLAR BONE GRAFTING

A key intervention prior to secondary alveolar bone grafting procedure is maxillary expansion. The primary objectives of maxillary expansion are to correct the transverse discrepancy (posterior cross-bite), establish the maxillary arch form, create room for alveolar bone graft placement by increasing the width of the alveolar cleft, and improve access to the alveolar bone graft area. Depending on the arch form and amount of relative anterior and posterior constrictions of the maxillary arch, either a differential expander (when more anterior expansion is required as opposed to posterior expansion) or a symmetric expander (when equal amounts of anterior and posterior expansions are required) may be used. For example, a maxillary arch that is collapsed in the canine area but without any cross-bite in the molar area would benefit from a differential expander as opposed to a symmetric expander. Various differential expanders are in vogue, but by far the most widely used one is the fan-shaped expander (**Fig. 18**). Hyrax- and Haas-type expanders with modifications are used for symmetric expansions. Quad helix appliances and their variants have also been widely used for maxillary expansion.[7,8] The authors recommend that maxillary expansion be initiated at least 6 months prior to the planned alveolar bone graft surgery.

Here are the key steps to do a differential maxillary expansion:

- Evaluate the dental casts to determine the relative amount of anterior versus posterior expansion. The magnitude of expansion is computed after placing the maxillary cast in a positive overjet relationship with the mandibular cast. If the mandibular molars are lingually tipped (compensations because of posterior cross-bite), the amount of tipping needs to be accounted for while computing the required maxillary expansion in the posterior segment.
- Ideally, 4 teeth (first permanent molars on each side if they have erupted into the arch are used as posterior abutments, and primary canines on each side are used as anterior abutments) with adequate root structure are selected for banding. Following adaptation of the bands, a pick-up impression is obtained for fabricating the expander. If maxillary first

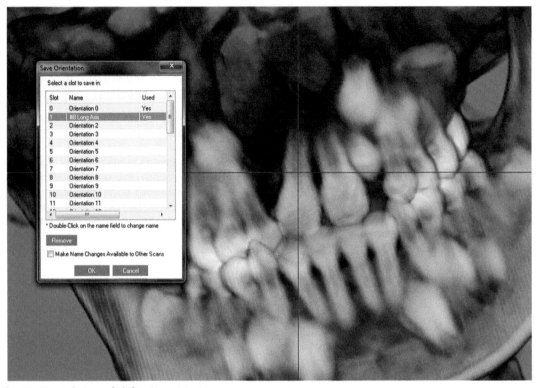

**Fig. 10.** Frontal view of cleft adjacent incisor.

permanent molars have not erupted sufficiently, then the maxillary second primary molars are banded and used as posterior abutments. Occasionally, it will be extremely difficult to place bands on the anterior abutment teeth because of the extremely collapsed maxillary anterior segment or malformed teeth. In such instances the authors recommend that the fan-shaped expander be modified to include mesial extension arms that are closely adapted to the palatal aspects of the anterior abutment teeth. Band cement or composite is used to bond the mesial extension arms to the anterior abutment teeth. This effectively serves as a 4-teeth banded expander.

**Fig. 11.** Lateral view of cleft adjacent incisor.

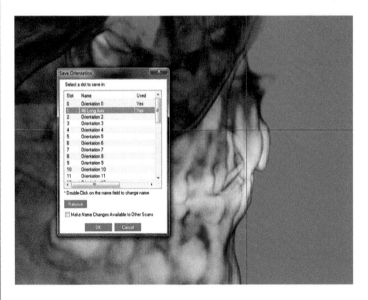

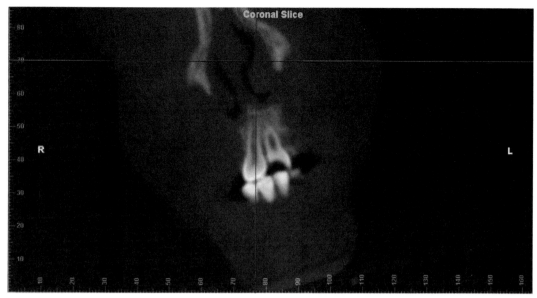

**Fig. 12.** Coronal slice of cleft adjacent incisor – adequate bone.

- The fulcrum of the appliance (differential maxillary expander) is designed to be placed at the appropriate location for the desired differential expansion ratio. The authors' laboratory experiments have suggested that a fulcrum placed 10 mm behind a line drawn from and to the central pits of the distal abutment teeth will yield an anterior-to-posterior expansion ratio of 1.95 to 1.[9] If the fulcrum is placed 7 mm behind the distal abutment, the anterior to posterior expansion ratio is 2.93 to 1. If the fulcrum is placed 5 mm behind the distal abutment, the anterior to posterior expansion ratio is 5.20 to 1. If the fulcrum is placed 3 mm behind the distal abutment, the anterior to posterior expansion is 27.33 to 1.[9]

- The appliance is cemented on the abutment teeth with band cement. The differential maxillary expansion appliance is activated by 1 turn every day until the maxillary arch is slightly overexpanded. Overexpansion is done to account for possible relapse. It has been the

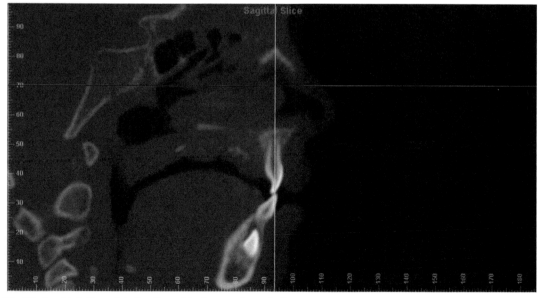

**Fig. 13.** Sagittal slice of cleft adjacent incisor – adequate bone.

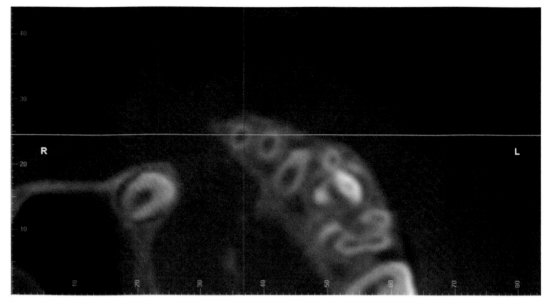

**Fig. 14.** Axial slice of cleft adjacent incisor near developing root apex – adequate bone.

authors' practice to overexpand by about 25%. Following this, the expansion screw of the appliance is sealed off with band cement to prevent any undesirable rotation of the expansion screw. Alternatively, a brass wire threaded through the activating screw will also suffice.

- Retention with a fixed transpalatal arch is recommended.

An ideal maxillary expansion outcome following use of a modified fan-shaped expansion appliance is presented in **Fig. 19**.

Determining the correct magnitude of expansion requires the team to predict and commit to the end-stage relationship between the maxillary and mandibular arches. This does not require deciding just how this relationship will be achieved but whether through functional appliance therapy, the use of Bollard plates, or via orthognathic surgery the decision taken to finish in a certain occlusion will allow for accurate expansion and reduced orthodontia during later stages of treatment.

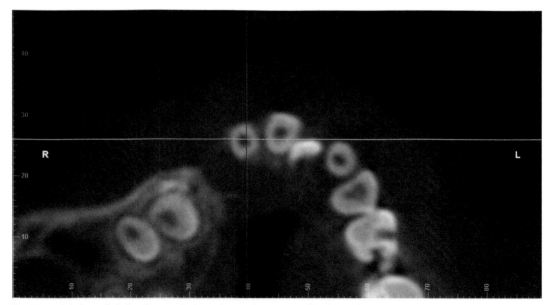

**Fig. 15.** Axial slice of cleft adjacent incisor nearer to crown – thin but adequate bone.

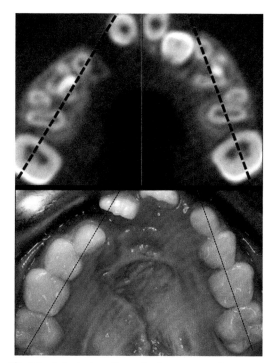

**Fig. 16.** Anteriorly collapsed minor segment.

## SUMMARY AND TAKE HOME POINTS
### What Are the Dento-Alveolar Effects of Rapid Maxillary Expansion in Children with Unilateral Complete Cleft Lip and Palate?

Ayub and colleagues[10] evaluated the effects of dento-alveolar effects of maxillary expansion in 25 children (9 girls and 16 boys) with unilateral complete cleft lip and palate and compared them with 27 children (13 girls and 14 boys) without any oro-facial clefts. Children with cleft lip and palate had their lip and palate repairs at 3 months and 12 months of age, respectively. Maxillary expansion was done using a Haas-type expander. Significant increases in maxillary transverse measurements, arch perimeters, palatal volumes, intermolar distance, and dental inclinations were observed in those with cleft lip and palate. Those with cleft lip and palate also experienced a decrease of arch length. These effects were similar in those without an oro-facial cleft.

The type of device that is best for cleft patients has been looked at by Figueiredo and colleagues,[11] who examined the dentoskeletal effects of 3 maxillary expanders in 30 patients divided into 3 groups. Using CBCT data, they confirmed the difference in anterior/posterior expansion when

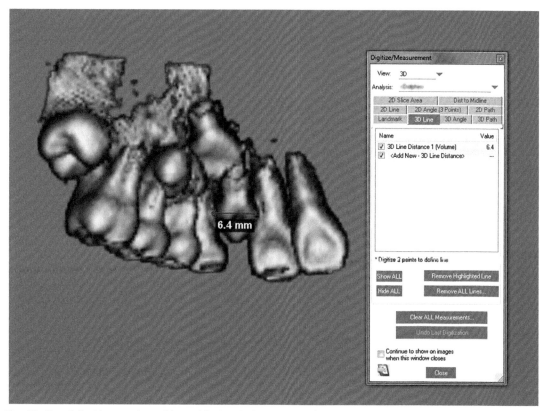

**Fig. 17.** Noncleft side peg-shaped lateral incisor being measured.

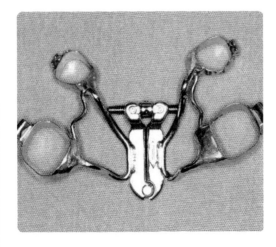

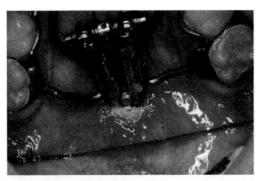

Fig. 20. Improperly placed fulcrum of appliance causing injury to palate.

of the supporting teeth as did the fan type.[11] Facanha and colleagues[12] compared symmetric Haas and Hyrax expanders in 48 children. They found no difference in the effect of the appliances using scanned casts to evaluate expansion at buccal cusp tips and the palatal cervical area of the teeth. In the authors' opinion, reliability and predictability of the outcome are most important. The fan expander may be modified to adapt to most clinical situations and offers these qualities.

### What Are Some Adverse Sequelae of Maxillary Expansion?

#### Injuries to surrounding tissues
While fabricating the appliance, utmost care should be taken to fit the bands appropriately and place the fulcrum in the desired position. The authors recommend that care providers pay considerable attention while trying the appliance in before cementing. Frequently, the fulcrum is placed behind the distal abutment, and there is a high likelihood of the fulcrum impinging on the palatal vault (Fig. 20).

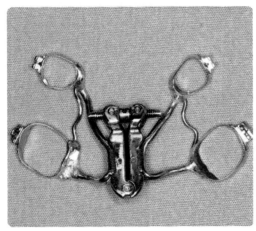

Fig. 18. Fan-shaped expander (differential maxillary expansion appliance).

symmetric (Hyrax) versus differential (fan and inverted minihyrax) were used. They also concluded that the inverted minihyrax optimized anterior expansion (no posterior expansion possible) without causing as much buccal tipping

#### Opening of palatal fistulas
One of the predicted sequelae of maxillary expansion is opening up of palatal fistulas. When a surgeon is dealing with a previously unrepaired fistula (Fig. 21A), the expansion of the fistula often facilitates better access for repair. In some cases of rapid maxillary expansion, a large fistula may result. In such scenarios, a 2-staged surgical procedure (closing of palatal fistula followed by alveolar bone grafting) may be required (Fig. 21B). Some orthodontists recommend slow expansion (1 turn every 3–4 days) to minimize the opening of large fistulas. The rationale for slow expansion is that there is time for the palatal tissues to adjust and adapt to the expansile stresses associated with maxillary expansion.

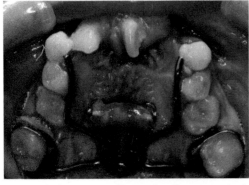

Fig. 19. Ideal expansion (3 months after expansion).

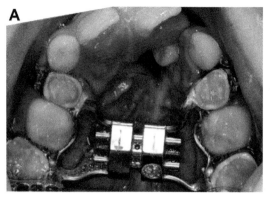
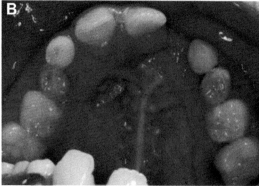

**Fig. 21.** (*A*) Oral-nasal fistula. (*B*) Two-staged surgery (palatal fistula repair followed by alveolar bone grafting).

### Traumatic occlusal forces in the bilateral cleft

Movement of the premaxilla, especially in the bilateral cleft patient, during masticatory function in the immediate postoperative period can substantially reduce the success of the bone graft. The orthodontist may be able to reduce these forces by positioning the teeth out of traumatic occlusion. The surgeon will also need to fabricate a maxillary interocclusal splint to reduce motion across the segments. Additionally, it may be necessary to surgically position the premaxilla out of traumatic occlusion by performing an osteotomy at the time of grafting.

### Relapse

This is by far the most commonly occurring sequela following maxillary expansion in those with complete cleft lip and palate. Because the midpalatal bone is missing, there is a high likelihood of collapse of the expanded maxillary shelves if appropriate retention protocols are not followed. The compressive stresses placed by the buccal musculature would be too high to be counteracted by a maxilla without palatal bone and collapse of the maxillary arch would occur rapidly without adequate retention. The appliance is maintained for at least 3 months after completion of expansion and thereafter retained with a fixed transpalatal arch or with orthodontic labial appliances (brackets with continuous arch wire) (**Figs. 22** and **23**). The authors recommend that the transpalatal arch be in place until the completion of the comprehensive phase of orthodontic treatment or at least until orthodontic labial appliances are placed.

### Improper arch form

Frequently, the maxillary anterior arch segments are collapsed and differential expansion is used to establish an ideal arch form. However, the differential expansion outcomes are not always predictable and would result in over expansion or establish an arch form that is, not compatible with the mandibular arch form.[13,14] Extreme care should be taken while designing the appliance and during activation to minimize this adverse sequelae.

### Is Orthodontic Treatment Always Required Following Alveolar Bone Grafting?

Although not always indicated, limited orthodontic treatment (usually in the maxillary arch) is done to facilitate eruption of permanent teeth into the arch following alveolar bone grafting. Usually the alveolar bone graft procedures are done no later than prior to eruption of maxillary permanent canines. For long-term success of alveolar bone grafts, physiologic stress needs to be placed on them.[15–17] This may be induced by either the permanent teeth erupting through the grafts or by moving the roots of adjacent permanent teeth into the grafted area. Orthodontic teeth movement may be started as soon as 8 weeks after alveolar bone graft procedure. However, the authors recommend that orthodontic teeth movement be

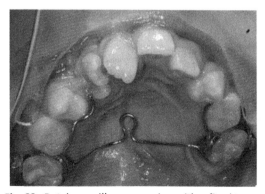

**Fig. 22.** Retain maxillary expansion with a fixed transpalatal arch.

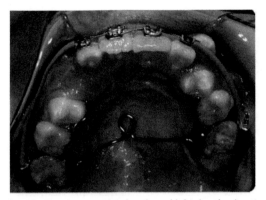

**Fig. 23.** Fixed transpalatal arch and labial orthodontic appliances for retaining maxillary expansion.

initiated following assurance of good bone quality in the grafted areas. This can be confirmed with radiographs. The authors recommend a 4- to 6-month waiting period following alveolar bone grafting to start orthodontic teeth movement. An ideal outcome is presented in **Fig. 24**A–D.

### Can Maxillary Expansion Be Done After Alveolar Bone Grafting Instead of Before Alveolar Bone Grafting?

Ideally, maxillary expansion needs to be done before alveolar bone grafting for the reasons outlined earlier. However in certain situations, the maxillary expansion is done following alveolar bone grafting. The rationale for doing the same is that arch expansion can serve as an effective

stimulator for regeneration of bone.[18–21] Uzel and colleagues[22] conducted a prospective clinical trial involving 30 patients with unilateral cleft lip and palate in the permanent dentition stage to examine the effects of maxillary expansion on late alveolar bone grafting. They found that bone graft volume loss was significantly lower in those who had maxillary expansion 6 weeks after secondary alveolar bone grafting when compared with those who had maxillary expansion before secondary alveolar bone grafting. Those who had maxillary expansion after the secondary alveolar bone grafting also had significantly higher increases in bone density 6 months after healing. However, there were no differences in mean graft volume and bone density between the 2 groups 12 months after the secondary alveolar bone graft. They concluded that maxillary expansion after secondary alveolar bone grafting could be a viable option in select cases with unilateral complete cleft lip and palate.

### Can Maxillary Expansion in Those with Cleft Lip and Plate Impact Root Development Process or Cause External Apical Root Resorption of Maxillary First Permanent Molars?

The maxillary expansion appliances usually use the first permanent molars as their posterior abutments, and clinicians are often concerned about the impact of stresses placed on the roots of abutment teeth during expansion. Cardinal and

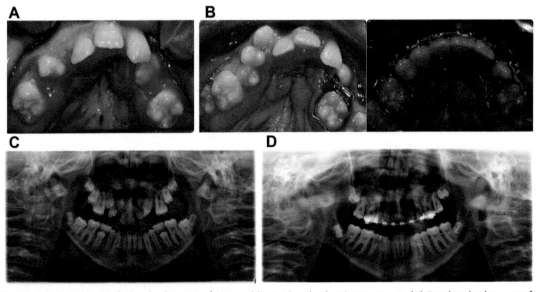

**Fig. 24.** Ideal outcome of alveolar bone grafting and limited orthodontic treatment. (A) Prealveolar bone grafting. (B) Postalveolar bone grafting and limited orthodontic treatment. (C) Prealveolar bone graft panoramic radiograph. (D) Postalveolar bone graft and limited orthodontic treatment panoramic radiograph.

colleagues[23] evaluated the impact of maxillary expansion on maxillary first permanent molar root morphology in subjects with unilateral cleft lip and palate. They evaluated the impact of using Hyrax, iMini, and fan type expanders on the root morphology.[23] Their results indicated that roots with open apexes had significant increases in root length after treatment, while those with closed apexes had no significant changes in root length, and they concluded that maxillary expansion does not inhibit the root development process or cause external apical root resorption.[23]

## DISCLOSURE

The authors have nothing to disclose.

## REFERENCES

1. Athanasiou AE, Mazaheri M, Zarrinnia K. Dental arch dimensions in patients with unilateral cleft-lip and palate. Cleft Palate J 1988;25:139–45.
2. Semb G. A study of facial growth in patients with unilateral cleft lip and palate treated by the Oslo CLP Team. Cleft Palate Craniofac J 1991;28:1–21.
3. Akcam MO, Toygar TU, Ozer L, et al. Evaluation of 3-dimensional tooth crown size in cleft lip and palate patients. Am J Orthod Dentofacial Orthop 2008; 134:85–92.
4. Antonarakis GS, Tompson BD, Fisher DM. Preoperative cleft lip measurements and maxillary growth in patients with unilateral cleft lip and palate. Cleft Palate Craniofac J 2016;53(6):e198–207.
5. Yoshida S, Suga K, Nakano Y, et al. Postoperative evaluation of grafted bone in alveolar cleft using three-dimensional computed tomography data. Cleft Palate Craniofac J 2013;50(6):671–7.
6. Vig K, Mercado K. Overview of orthodontic care for children with cleft lip and palate, 1915-2015. Am J Orthod Dentofacial Orthop 2015;148:543–56.
7. Aizenbud D, Hazan-Molina H, Peled M, et al. The reverse quad helix expander: easy access for bone graft manipulation in the cleft maxilla. Pediatr Dent 2013;35(4):120–3.
8. Aizenbud D, Ciceu C, Rachmiel A, et al. Reverse quad helix appliance: differential anterior maxillary expansion of the cleft area before bone grafting. J Craniofac Surg 2012;23(5):e440–3.
9. Bruun R, Shusterman S, Nison M. An effective means of differential palatal expansion in cleft lip and palate patients. A paper in satisfaction of research requirements at HSDM. March 1994.
10. Ayub PV, Janson G, Gribel BF, et al. Analysis of the maxillary dental arch after rapid maxillary expansion in patients with unilateral complete cleft lip and palate. Am J Orthod Dentofacial Orthop 2016;149(5): 705–15.
11. Figueiredo D, Bartolomeo F, Romualdo C, et al. Dentoskeletal effects of 3 maxillary expanders in patients with clefts: a cone-beam computed tomography study. Am J Orthod Dentofacial Orthop 2014;146:73–81.
12. Facanha A, Lara T, Garib D, et al. Transverse effect of Haas and Hyrax appliances on the upper dental arch in patients with unilateral complete cleft lip and palate: a comparative study. Dental Press J Orthod 2014;19(2):39–45.
13. Pan X, Qian Y, Yu J, et al. Biomechanical effects of rapid palatal expansion on the craniofacial skeleton with cleft palate: a three-dimensional finite element analysis. Cleft Palate Craniofac J 2007; 44:149–54.
14. Wang D, Cheng L, Wang C, et al. Biomechanical analysis of rapid maxillary expansion in the UCLP patient. Med Eng Phys 2009;31:409–17.
15. Eppley BL, Sadove AM. Management of alveolar cleft bone grafting—state of art. Cleft Palate Craniofac J 2000;;37:229.
16. Guo J, Li C, Zhang Q, et al. Secondary bone grafting for alveolar cleft in children with cleft lip or cleft lip and palate. Cochrane Database Syst Rev 2011;(6): CD008050.
17. Semb G. Alveolar bone grafting. Front Oral Biol 2012;;16:124.
18. Bergland O, Semb G, Abyholm F. Elimination of the residual alveolar cleft by secondary bone grafting and subsequent orthodontic treatment. Cleft Palate J 1986;;23:175.
19. Boyne PJ, Sands NR. Combined orthodontic-surgical management of residual palato-alveolar cleft defects. Am J Orthod 1976;;70:20.
20. Cavassan Ade O, de Albuquerque MD, Filho LC. Rapid maxillary expansion after secondary alveolar bone graft in a patient with bilateral cleft lip and palate. Cleft Palate Craniofac J 2004;;4:333.
21. Da Silva Filho OG, Boiani E, Cavassan AO, et al. Rapid maxillary expansion after secondary alveolar bone grafting in patients with alveolar cleft. Cleft Palate Craniofac J 2009;;46:331.
22. Uzel A, Benlidayı ME, Kürkçü M, et al. The effects of maxillary expansion on late alveolar bone grafting in patients with unilateral cleft lip and palate. J Oral Maxillofac Surg 2019;77(3):607–14.
23. Cardinal L, da Rosa Zimermann G, Mendes FM, et al. The impact of rapid maxillary expansion on maxillary first molar root morphology of cleft subjects. Clin Oral Investig 2018;22(1):369–76.

# Obturation and Tissue Transfer for Large Craniofacial Defects

Curtis D. Schmidt, DDS, Stavan Y. Patel, DDS, MD*,
Jennifer E. Woerner, DMD, MD, Ghali E. Ghali, DDS, MD, FRCS(Ed)

### KEYWORDS

- Craniofacial • Reconstruction • Prosthetic obturator • Obturation • Tissue transfer

### KEY POINTS

- Reconstruction of craniofacial defects should be individualized to each patient and defect.
- Reconstructive goals should be prioritized and should be kept in mind when deciding on an ideal reconstructive option.
- Given the complexity of the craniofacial anatomy and functional demand, tissue transfer is considered preferentially over traditional prosthetic obturation for reconstruction of large craniofacial defects.
- Obturation using a dentofacial prosthesis is a viable option for reconstruction of small maxillary and midface defects in select patients.
- Patient motivation, meticulous hygiene, and long-term follow-up are important for maintenance and success of the obturator prosthesis.

## INTRODUCTION

The elegant and detailed anatomy of the craniofacial and stomatognathic complex is both unique and critical to life-sustaining functions. The calvarium and the bones of the upper face house and protect not only the motherboard of the central nervous system but also the exclusive critical elements for the senses of sight, sound, taste, and smell. The bones and soft tissue of the lower face make possible not only deglutition and phonation but maintain the entry point for respiration as well as its sense of taste.

When portions of this highly evolved system are lost reconstruction is critical, given the connected and supportive nature of the entire complex. The ideal reconstruction is therefore potentially very complex. Underlying deep elements of the reconstruction, such as bony and cartilaginous structures not externally visible, must have the strength and integrity to support overlying soft tissues and housed organs or tissues such as the eyes and the teeth. Visible elements of the reconstruction must have appropriate contours, plasticity, color, and range of motion to restore connection, confluence, and esthetics. The ideal reconstruction would also be inexpensive, effective, durable, and maintenance free, and would restore integrity between anatomic cavities while also eliminating pathologic cavities. Ideally, these goals could be accomplished with minimal host morbidity through the harvest of autogenous tissues. The ideal reconstruction must also consider factors such as the tolerance of the patient to

Department of Oral and Maxillofacial Surgery/Head and Neck Surgery, Louisiana State University Health Sciences Center, 1501 Kings Highway, Shreveport, LA 71103, USA
* Corresponding author.
*E-mail address:* spate9@lsuhsc.edu

Oral Maxillofacial Surg Clin N Am 32 (2020) 219–232
https://doi.org/10.1016/j.coms.2020.01.009

**Table 1**
**Functional reconstructive goals based on head and neck units**

| Unit | Subunits | Functional Goals of Reconstruction |
|---|---|---|
| Head | Cranium, scalp | Provide bony continuity<br>Avoid exposure of cranial bone<br>Keep intracranial contents isolated |
| Midface | Nose, eyes, ears, cheek, maxilla, skull base | Nasal breathing<br>Patent auditory canal<br>Globe position<br>Unrestricted globe movement<br>Unobstructed vision<br>Eyelid competency<br>Avoid entropion or ectropion<br>Intelligible speech<br>Mastication<br>Separate sinuses<br>Isolate intracranial components |
| Lower face | Mandible, lips | Unrestricted temporomandibular<br>  joint mobility<br>Stable occlusion<br>Diet<br>Mastication<br>Intelligible speech<br>Lip competency<br>Avoid microstomia<br>Unrestricted mouth opening |
| Oral cavity | Tongue, floor of mouth, palate, buccal mucosa, dentition | Intelligible speech<br>Swallowing<br>Provide alimentary tract<br>Isolation of oral cavity from sinuses<br>  and nasal cavity<br>Unrestricted mouth opening<br>Avoid aspiration<br>Mastication<br>Diet<br>Stable occlusion |
| Neck | Pharynx, larynx, esophagus | Provide alimentary tract<br>Stable airway<br>Functional swallowing<br>Avoid aspiration<br>Intelligible speech<br>Protect great vessels |

prolonged surgical procedures, the patient's financial situation, life expectancy, and personal desires.

One viable option when considering these limitations is traditional prosthetic obturation. Although prosthetic obturation is generally viewed as a conciliatory reconstruction, it is often necessary because of patients' systematic factors, the nature of the tissue loss, or other social constraints. Aside from scholarly definitions of obturation, in the surgical community obturation is generally understood to be not only a method of eliminating communication between 2 anatomic or pathologic cavities but is also generally understood to fill some other role relating to tissue loss. Although obturation is unlikely, if not impossible, to meet all of the ideal reconstructive goals in head and neck reconstruction, a well-executed obturation still has the potential to accomplish many of these goals. A myriad of acrylics, metals, and other advanced materials are now available at the hands of a skilled prosthetist. Alternatively, tissue can be transferred locally, regionally, or remotely to obturate defects, or allogeneic or autogenetic tissues can be grafted.

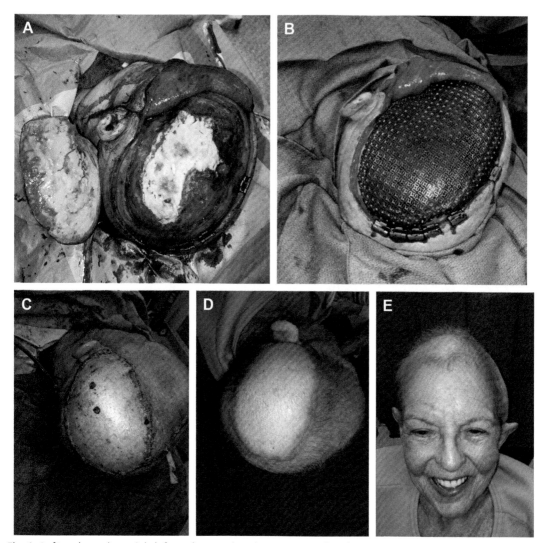

**Fig. 1.** Left scalp and cranial defect obturated and reconstructed with a myocutaneous latissimus dorsi free flap. (*A*) Extensive defect of the scalp with underlying necrotic bone flap and associated supradural infection. (*B*) Cranial bone resected to healthy bleeding bone and reconstructed with titanium mesh. (*C*) Latissimus dorsi free flap inset and wound closure. (*D, E*) Three-month follow-up photos showing viability of the flap, maintenance of the cranial integrity, good form, and overall improvement in patient's quality of life.

When comparing a material-driven or prosthetic obturation with a tissue-driven obturation, the most glaring difference is the fixed versus removable nature of the obturation. A material fabricated obturator must be removed and able to be easily cleaned and reinserted by the patient. Although it has the potential to have a near perfect color match, it does not have the potential to change color in response to sun and aging as the rest of the patient's skin is likely to do. A material obturator, in addition to having the potential of breakage and fatigue, is unlikely to last for the entire life of the patient and will likely need to be recreated. A material obturator often has the ability, through serial adjustments, to decrease the size of the communication intended to be obturated. Although a tissue-based reconstruction contrasts each of these characteristics, it usually involves donor-site morbidity, potential for tissue thickness, color and texture mismatch, longer hospital stays, and multiple trips to the operating room. Furthermore, lack of reach of local and pedicled flaps and a vessel-depleted neck may make distant tissue transfer challenging. Cost comparisons are difficult to make and involve complicated calculations such as fees of the

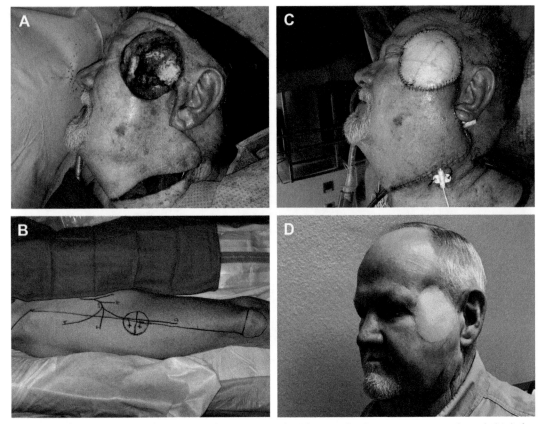

**Fig. 2.** Left skull base defect obturated and reconstructed with a myofasciocutaneous anterolateral thigh free flap. (*A*) Extent of the skull base, preauricular and total parotidectomy defect. (*B*) Right anterolateral thigh free flap anatomic and vascular markings. (*C*) Anterolateral thigh free flap inset and wound closure. (*D*) One-year follow-up photo after adjuvant radiation, showing flap with skin color mismatch but maintaining integrity and bulk at the skull base.

prosthetist and materials, potential need for refabrication, surgical time, length of hospital stays, and cost of any required medications over the life of the obturation.

Regardless of the type of obturation chosen, it can be both a challenging and rewarding endeavor for both the surgeon and the patient, and most

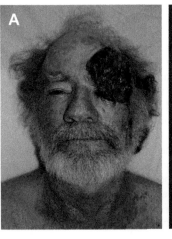

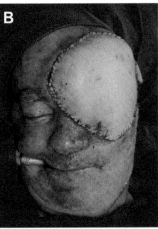

**Fig. 3.** Left orbital obturation and facial skin reconstruction with a myofasciocutaneous anterolateral thigh free flap. (*A*) Left eyebrow and upper eyelid cutaneous squamous cell carcinoma with involvement of the globe and orbital content. (*B*) After tumor resection and after orbital exenteration defect was obturated and reconstructed with an anterolateral thigh free flap.

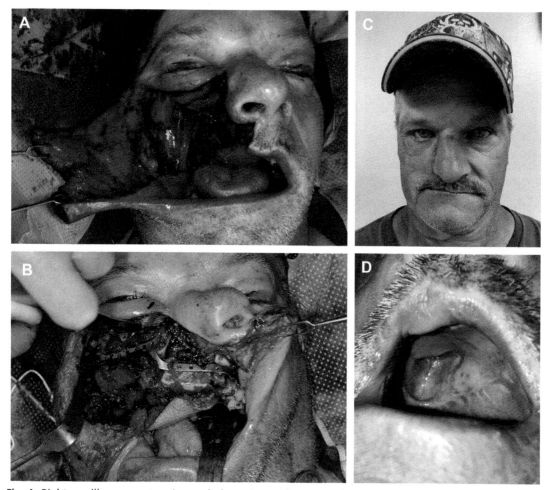

**Fig. 4.** Right maxillary reconstruction and obturation with an osteofasciocutaneous fibula free flap. (*A*) Right hemi-maxillectomy defect involving the right zygoma, and orbital rim and floor. (*B*) Reconstruction of the orbital floor and rim, inset of the three-segment fibula, and complex reconstruction of the palate and the maxillary/labial vestibules with the adjoining skin paddle. (*C, D*) One-year postoperative clinical photos after adjuvant radiation showing fair projection and esthetics of the right cheek and upper lip, maintenance of good lip function, and obturation of the palatomaxillary defect.

often is a decision that should be made after careful discussion between surgeon and patient.

## GOALS OF RECONSTRUCTION

The goals of reconstruction should be individualized to each patient's needs, but have to be prioritized for maintenance of integrity of craniofacial tissue, improving function, and restoration of form, while minimizing morbidity to the patient and improving his or her quality of life.[1] The individualization of goals to patients should take into account their health, comorbidities, body habitus, and wishes. Maintenance of integrity of the craniofacial components is of paramount importance, followed by restoration of function and form. Restoration of form includes recreation of craniofacial contour, consistency (texture, color, bulkiness), and dimensions (width, height, projection). **Table 1** illustrates various different functional reconstructive goals based on various craniofacial subunits.[1]

## RECONSTRUCTIVE OPTIONS

For a given craniofacial defect, the ideal reconstructive option is based on several considerations, which include patient-related factors, type of craniofacial defect, the surgical team's experience and expertise, availability of appropriate surgical tools and facilities, and reconstructive goals.[1] Patient-related factors such as

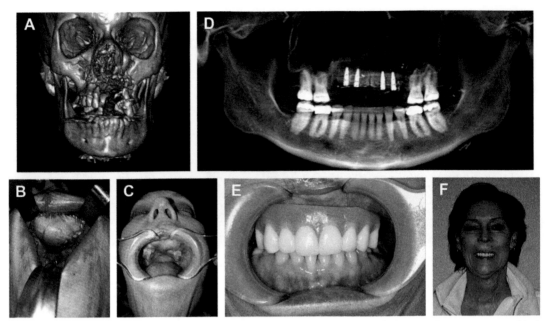

**Fig. 5.** Post-traumatic palatal and anterior maxillary defect reconstructed with an osteofasciocutaneous fibula free flap. (*A*) A three-dimensional rendering of computed tomography scan at presentation showing the maxillary and palatal bony defects caused after a high-velocity ballistic injury. (*B*) Surgical site post reconstruction of maxilla with 2 fibula segments and obturation of oronasal fistula with the skin paddle from the fibula free flap. (*C*) Four-month postoperative view of the skin paddle and surgical site. (*D*) Orthopantomogram showing integration of fibula into the native maxilla and tertiary reconstruction of the defect with 4 osseointegrated implants. (*E*, *F*) One-year postoperative results showing restoration of dentition, facial form, lip projection and function, and improved quality of life.

comorbidities, body habitus, survival prognosis, and history of irradiation or future plans for adjuvant radiation should be given significant thought before deciding on the ideal reconstructive options. It is important to consider all of these along with patients' wishes and family support, as these factors can affect reconstruction options

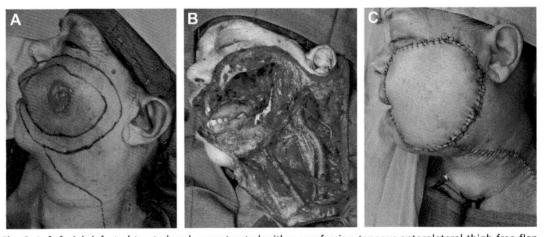

**Fig. 6.** Left facial defect obturated and reconstructed with a myofasciocutaneous anterolateral thigh free flap. (*A*) Buccal mucosal squamous cell carcinoma with involvement of the adjacent skin and lip. (*B*) After composite resection of the tissues affected by the malignancy and modified radical neck dissection. (*C*) Anterolateral thigh free flap inset and wound closure with effective obturation of the facial defect, providing for maintenance of integrity and coverage of exposed great vessels in the neck, and reconstructing the contour and facial form.

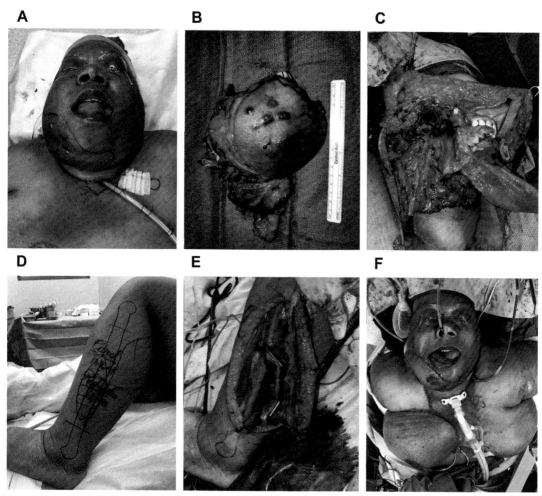

**Fig. 7.** Right facial and mandibular defect obturated and reconstructed with a left osteofasciocutaneous fibula free flap and a right myocutaneous pectoralis major pedicled flap. (*A*) Advanced mandibular squamous cell carcinoma with involvement of the adjacent skin, nodal metastasis, and acute hemorrhage from the tumor site. (*B*) Specimen from tumor extirpation and right modified radical neck dissection. (*C*) Surgical defect after composite resection of hemi-mandible and floor of mouth, partial glossectomy, infrastructure maxillectomy, and right pharyngectomy. (*D*) Left lower extremity with fibula free flap and vascular markings. (*E*) Donor-site anatomy with harvested fibula free flap skin paddle and 3 segments of fibula bone adapted to a transosseous reconstruction plate. (*F*) Immediate postoperative photo showing intraoral defect lined with the fibula flap skin paddle and the facial skin defect supplemented with the pectoralis major flap skin paddle. Because of the extent of the defect, both flaps were necessary to effectively obturate the orofacial communication.

(prosthetic obturation versus tissue transfer) and/or flap selection.

Flap selection for a particular defect is complex, but briefly it should be based on accurate preoperative prediction of defect size, depth, location, and type of tissue needed for reconstruction. Given the extensive availability of various nonvascularized grafts, local flaps, regional flaps, and distant donor site (free flaps), and advances in anatomic knowledge and surgical technology, nowadays prosthetic obturation is not always an ideal

reconstructive option for every patient and each craniofacial defect, especially in an irradiated field. Historically, prosthetic obturation was advantageous because of its benefits of oncologic surveillance, shorter operative time, and shorter hospital stay, and was primarily used for reconstruction of small maxillary or midface defects. However, given its drawbacks of lack of patient compliance, need for routine maintenance, difficulties with hygiene, removal, cleaning, and replacement of prosthesis, and poor quality of life when compared with defects

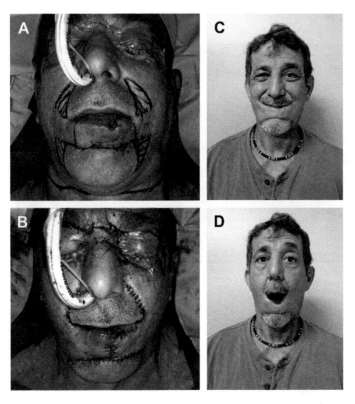

**Fig. 8.** Lower lip squamous cell carcinoma resection and reconstruction with local flaps. (*A*) Lower lip malignancy with marked resection margins and markings for a Bernard-Burow flap with Webster modification, which is to be used for reconstruction of the lower lip defect. (*B*) Flap advancement post resection, and inset photograph showing good lip length and competency. (*C, D*) Six-week postoperative photos showing good lip function in smile and mouth opening. The patient was able to tolerate a regular diet by mouth without any significant concerns.

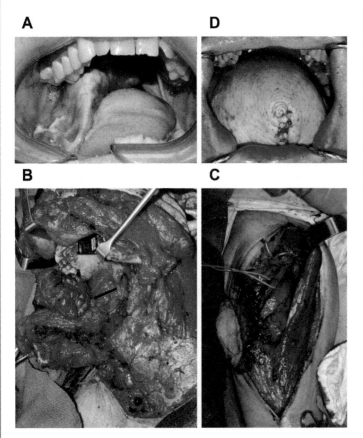

**Fig. 9.** Subtotal glossectomy and floor of mouth defect obturated and reconstructed with a right myofasciocutaneous anterolateral thigh free flap. (*A*) Intraoral photo showing the aggressive neoplasm, a recurrent sarcomatoid variant of squamous cell carcinoma. (*B*) Photograph showing subtotal resection of the tongue, floor of mouth, and right mandible. (*C*) Harvest of the anterolateral thigh free flap. (*D*) Anterolateral thigh free flap inset into the defect to recreate the tongue mound and obturate the floor of mouth.

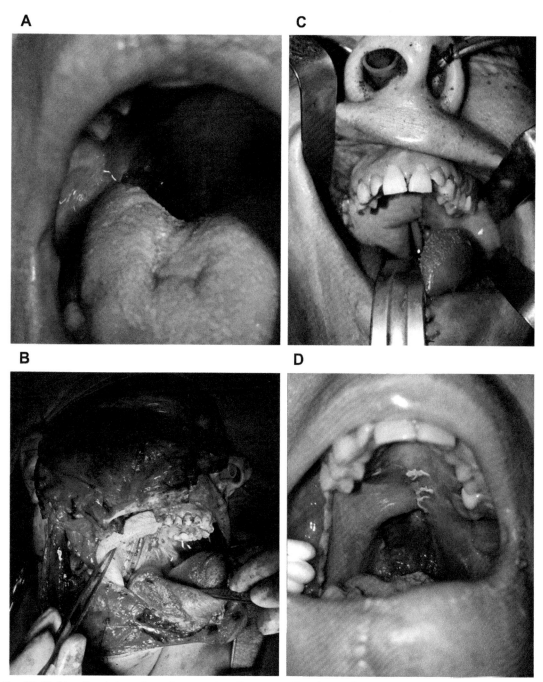

**Fig. 10.** Right soft palate and oropharyngeal malignancy extirpation and reconstruction with a fasciocutaneous radial forearm free flap. (*A*) Clinical photo showing the tumor involving the right soft palate, palatoglossal arch, and the glossotonsillar sulcus. (*B*) Lip-split mandibular osteotomy performed to access the lesion. Photo showing post–tumor extirpation status and modified radial neck dissection defect with complex folding and inset of the radial forearm free flap. (*C*) Intraoperative view of the flap inset into the palate, lateral pharynx, and base of tongue. (*D*) One-month postoperative photo of the reconstructed oropharynx.

reconstructed with free tissue transfer and implant-supported overdenture,[2,3] its use has been pushed further to the end of the reconstructive algorithm. Furthermore, it is not an ideal reconstructive option in an irradiated field because of the risk of osteoradionecrosis, and not all defects such as cranial (**Fig. 1**), skull base (**Fig. 2**), orbital (**Fig. 3**), maxillary (**Figs. 4** and **5**), cheek (**Fig. 6**), mandibular (**Fig. 7**),

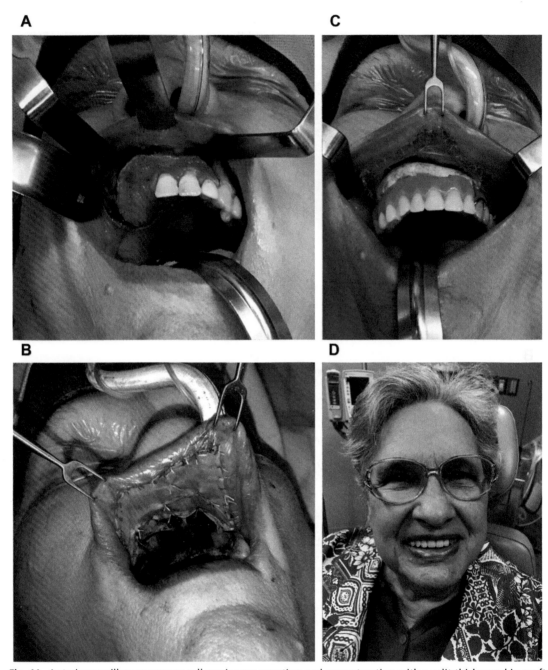

**Fig. 11.** Anterior maxillary squamous cell carcinoma resection and reconstruction with a split-thickness skin graft and a traditional maxillary obturator. (*A*) Photo showing tumor resection margins. (*B*) Post resection maxillary defect with the excised mucosa being lined with a split-thickness skin graft. (*C*) Placement of an immediate traditional obturator that is being retained by the remaining palate, left maxillary dentition, and right maxillary edentulous alveolar ridge. (*D*) Three-month postoperative photograph showing good esthetic outcome, with the patient being able retain the prosthesis with minimal nasal regurgitation and speech impediment.

lip (**Fig. 8**), floor of mouth and tongue (**Fig. 9**), and oropharyngeal (**Fig. 10**) defects can be reconstructed with a traditional prosthetic obturator. At the authors' institution, tissue transfer (local, regional, or distant flaps) is given primary consideration over prosthetic obturation. The only time a prosthesis is given priority over tissue transfer is when in select patients their health, comorbidities, body habitus, prognosis, or wishes do not allow for tissue transfer. For these patients, a

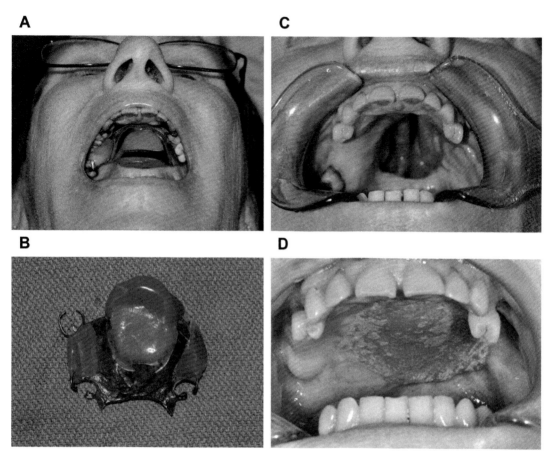

**Fig. 12.** Oronasal fistula obturation and palatal reconstruction with a fasciocutaneous radial forearm free flap. (*A*) Patient at presentation; using a traditional obturator to prevent communication between mouth and sinonasal cavities. The obturator is being supported by the existing anterior and right maxillary dentition. (*B*) Clinical photo of the obturator showing the clasps used to retain the prosthesis and the palatal bulb used to prevent passage of air, saliva, and food into the sinonasal cavities. (*C*) Clinical photo of the patient without the obturator, showing the extent of palatal defect. (*D*) Three-month postoperative photo showing palatal reconstruction, healed radial forearm free flap, and obturated oronasal fistula.

traditional prosthetic obturator can be used to reconstruct a partial maxillectomy or smaller palatal defects with appropriate bony and soft-tissue support (**Fig. 11**). Having appropriate support is necessary for retention and stability of the obturator. They can also be used to temporarily obturate oronasal or oroantral fistulas (**Fig. 12**), prevent food regurgitation, or improve speech in growing children for whom tissue transfer is not appropriate or an available option. When tissue transfer is a viable option in patients with developmental and congenital anomalies, it should be preferentially considered over other less reliable conservative surgical modalities (**Figs. 13–15**).

During planning for reconstruction of large craniofacial defects, traditional prosthetic obturation is generally not given much consideration as a viable reconstructive option. For large defects, reconstruction should be tailored to each individual craniofacial subunit. Consideration should be given to type and volume of tissue needed for ideal reconstruction. Ideal flaps used for obturation of extensive craniofacial defects would provide for large skin surface with good color match, sufficient tissue volume, long and consistent vascular pedicle, and minimal donor-site morbidity (**Fig. 16**). Flaps harvested from the arm, chest, back, abdomen, and thigh regions provide most of the characteristics needed for soft-tissue reconstruction of large defects. These flaps can then be used with other flaps such as the fibula and scapula free flaps for reconstruction of the bony contour and defects. Pedicled pectoralis major and latissimus dorsi flaps, and free fibula, scapula, radial forearm, and anterolateral thigh flaps are considered the ideal flaps for reconstruction and obturation of extensive craniofacial defects.

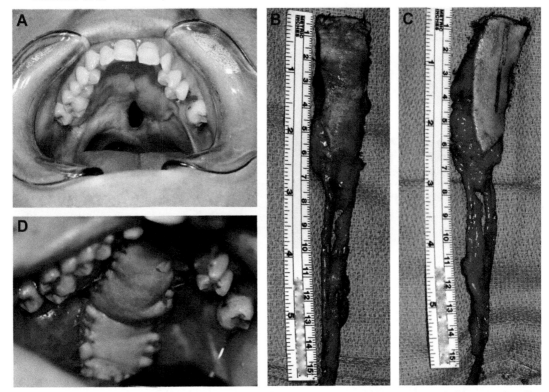

**Fig. 13.** Oronasal fistula and soft palate reconstruction with a laminated fasciocutaneous radial forearm free flap. (*A*) Patient with history of cleft palate with repeated attempts at repair and pharyngoplasty, continues to have significant scarring of the mucosa, persistent oronasal fistula and velopharyngeal insufficiency. (*B–C*) Harvest of a radial forearm free flap and its lamination with split thickness skin graft. (*D*) Inset of flap into the palatal defect to obturate the oronasal fistula and reconstruct the oropharynx.

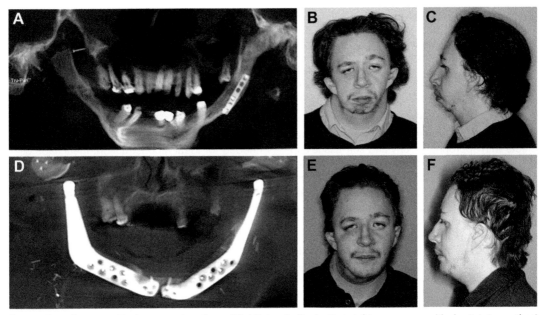

**Fig. 14.** Complete mandibular reconstruction with bilateral alloplastic total temporomandibular joint prosthesis and fibula free flap. (*A*) Orthopantomogram of a patient with Nager Syndrome, who was previously treated with repeated mandibular distraction osteogenesis and bone grafting. Radiograph showing poor bony support for existing dentition, retained hardware at the right skull base and left temporomandibular joint ankylosis. (*B, C*) Clinical photographs of the patient at the time of presentation. (*D*) Postoperative orthopantomogram of the same patient after total mandibulectomy, removal of foreign body, release of left temporomandibular joint ankylosis and reconstruction with bilateral total joints and a three segment fibula free flap. (*E, F*) Six month postoperative photos showing improved form and facial projection.

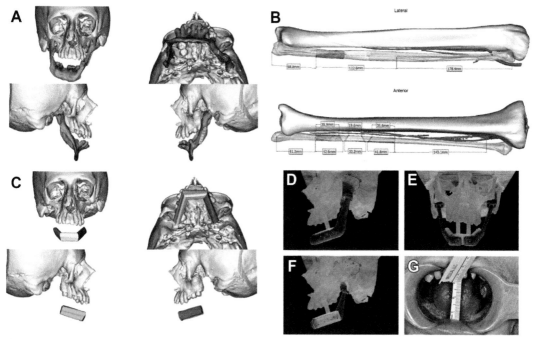

**Fig. 15.** Surgical planning for total mandibular reconstruction with custom joints and free tissue transfer, same patient from figure 14. (*A*) A three-dimensional rendering of computed tomography scan at presentation. (*B*) Planning for fibula bone harvest. (*C*) Virtual removal of mandible and plan for three segment fibula free flap. (*D-F*) Creation of stereolithographic skull/fibula model, designing and fabrication of custom alloplastic temporomandibular joint prosthesis. (*G*) Final outcome at three month postoperative visit showing good mouth opening and function.

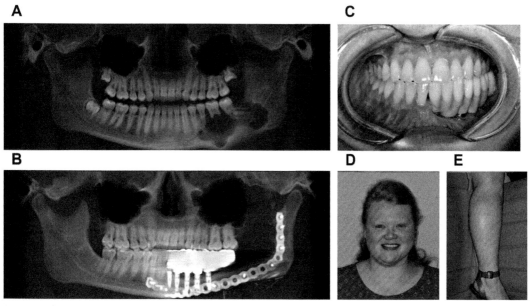

**Fig. 16.** Left mandibular tumor resection and reconstruction with a right osseous fibula free flap. (*A*) Orthopantomogram showing left mandibular benign odontogenic tumor. (*B*) Orthopantomogram of the same patient 10 years after resection of the tumor and reconstruction with a 2-segment fibula free flap, placement of transosseous reconstruction plate, and a 5-osseointegrated implant-supported prosthesis. (*C–E*) Long-term clinical photos showing stability and esthetics of the dental prosthesis and minimal donor-site morbidity at the right lower extremity flap harvest site.

## SUMMARY

Reconstruction and obturation of craniomaxillofacial defects is certainly a complex and challenging topic. For extensive craniofacial defects, the use of locoregional flaps and free tissue transfer is likely the ideal way of obturating these defects. That being said, for small to moderate-size maxillary defects involving dentition and in specific patient populations, the use of a traditional prosthetic obturator would be beneficial and should be considered as a viable reconstructive option.

## DISCLOSURE

The authors have nothing to disclose.

## REFERENCES

1. Patel SY, Meram AT, Kim DD. Soft tissue reconstruction for head and neck ablative defects. Oral Maxillofac Surg Clin North Am 2019;31(1):39–68.

2. Kumar VV, Jacob PC, Ebenezer S, et al. Implant supported dental rehabilitation following segmental mandibular reconstruction- quality of life outcomes of a prospective randomized trial. J Cranio Maxillofac Surg 2016;44(7):800–10.

3. Brandão TB, Vechiato J, Eduardo V, et al. Obturator prostheses versus free tissue transfers: a systematic review of the optimal approach to improving the quality of life for patients with maxillary defects. J Prosthet Dent 2016;115(2):247–53.

# An Overview of Craniosynostosis Craniofacial Syndromes for Combined Orthodontic and Surgical Management

Shayna Azoulay-Avinoam, DDS[a], Richard Bruun, DDS[b],
James MacLaine, BDS[c], Veerasathpurush Allareddy, BDS, PhD[a],*,
Cory M. Resnick, DMD, MD[d], Bonnie L. Padwa, DMD, MD[e]

## KEYWORDS

- Craniosynostosis • Maxillary distraction osteogenesis • Craniofacial syndromes • Apert syndrome
- Pfieffer syndrome • Crouzon syndrome

## KEY POINTS

- Patients with craniosynostosis syndromes require comprehensive multidisciplinary care.
- Common presenting clinical features include maxillary hypoplasia, class III malocclusions, anterior openbites.
- Excellent outcomes can be achieved with good teamwork.

## OVERVIEW OF CRANIOSYNOSTOSIS

Craniosynostosis, defined as the premature fusion of 1 or more cranial sutures, occurs in 1 in 2000 to 2500 live births and is one of the most common congenital craniofacial anomalies.[1–3] Lack of growth perpendicular to the fused sutures and compensatory growth at normal ones result[4–6] in patients presenting with a distorted head shape. Most cases of craniosynostosis are isolated or nonsyndromic, but 9% to 40% of patients have a syndromic form with more than 130 syndromes associated with craniosynostois.[6–9] Patients with syndromic craniosynostosis may also have associated abnormalities of the face, trunk, and extremities that vary in presentation, severity, and cause.[3,4,6–9] Early diagnosis and treatment of craniosynostosis is important to ensure that brain growth is not restricted by insufficient cranial volume and to minimize distortion of the cranium. In severe cases, affected patients may have increased intracranial pressure (ICP) and experience functional problems (eg, breathing difficulty, choking or vomiting with feeding), exorbitism, irritability, developmental delays, and even death.[4,10,11]

Funding: This report was supported in part by an American Association of Orthodontists Foundation Research Aid Award to Dr S. Azoulay-Avinoam.

[a] Department of Orthodontics, College of Dentistry, University of Illinois at Chicago, 801 South Paulina Street, 138AD (MC841), Chicago, IL 60612-7211, USA; [b] Boston Children's Hospital Cleft Lip/Palate and Craniofacial Teams, Department of Dentistry, Boston Children's Hospital, Harvard School of Dental Medicine, 300 Longwood Avenue, Boston, MA 02115, USA; [c] Department of Developmental Biology, Boston Children's Hospital, Harvard School of Dental Medicine, 300 Longwood Avenue, Boston, MA 02115, USA; [d] Oral & Maxillofacial Surgery Program, Department of Plastic & Oral Surgery, Harvard Medical School, 300 Longwood Avenue, Hunnewell, 1st Floor, Boston, MA 02115, USA; [e] Section of Oral and Maxillofacial Surgery, Department of Plastic & Oral Surgery, Harvard Medical School, 300 Longwood Avenue, Hunnewell, 1st Floor, Boston, MA 02115, USA
* Corresponding author.
E-mail address: sath@uic.edu

## EPIDEMIOLOGY

Several studies have investigated the incidence and prevalence of craniosynostosis across different regions.[1,3] In Western Australia, prevalence of craniosynostosis between the years of 1980 and 1994 was 5.06 per 10,000 births, similar to the prevalence of 4.3 per 10,000 in the metro-Atlanta area from 1989 to 2003.[1,3] The Agency for Healthcare Research and Quality Healthcare Cost and Utilization Project Kids Inpatient Database estimates prevalence of craniosynostosis at 3.5 to 4.5 per 10,000 births between 1997 and 2006.[12] These values are lower than those from other studies in regions such as Colorado (14.1 per 10,000), New South Wales (8.1 per 10,000), and Israel (6.0 per 10,000) for a coincident time period.[1,13,14] The same study in Australia showed an increase in lambdoid synostosis of 15.7% per year linearly and did not distinguish a particular cause or explanation.[1] In contrast, its metro-Atlanta counterpart discovered a decrease in prevalence of lambdoid synostosis and attributed this to a possible misclassification of deformational posterior plagiocephaly in these patients.[3]

## SYNDROMIC VERSUS NONSYNDROMIC CRANIOSYNOSTOSIS

The diagnosis of, risk factors associated with, and management of nonsyndromic or syndromic craniosynostosis syndromes differ markedly. Among the nonsyndromic population, sagittal synostosis is the most common, followed by synostosis of the lambdoid suture, whereas coronal suture involvement is more characteristic of syndromic craniosynostosis.[1] Boulet and colleagues[3] found that 39% of nonsyndromic cases had sagittal synostosis and that this was more common in boys, whereas coronal synostosis was more common in girls. Being male is also a risk factor for lambdoid synostosis. Although less severe, other major birth defects were still noted in 11.2% of nonsyndromic patients.[1] Syndromic craniosynostosis is more complex, harder to care for, and necessitates multidisciplinary treatment. It is also associated with an increased risk of increased ICP caused by intracranial venous congestion, hydrocephalus, and upper airway obstruction.[9] Syndromic patients are at the greatest risk for perioperative complications.[15] Diagnosis of a syndrome is based primarily on dysmorphologic presentation and genetic testing, and, according to Singer and colleagues,[1] 25.3% of patients with craniosynostosis are seen by a geneticist.[10]

## GENETICS

Johnson and Wilkie[8] reported that 21% of patients with craniosynostosis had a genetic diagnosis of single-gene mutations or chromosomal abnormalities. Craniosynostosis is mostly autosomal dominant and is more likely to be associated with multiple-suture synostosis and extracranial complications. The most common mutations are in the FGFR2, FGFR3, TWIST1, and EFNB1 genes.[8] Crouzon, Apert, and Pfeiffer syndromes are caused by mutation to the FGFR-2 gene, Saethre-Chotzen is caused by the TWIST-1 gene mutation, and Muenke is unique in that there is a mutation in the FGFR-3 gene.[9,16–19] In a study by Timberlake and Persing,[20] exome sequencing was completed in 384 families and a new genetic testing protocol was established. It had been previously determined that syndromic craniosynostoses are associated with mutations in the FGF/Ras/ERK, BMP, Wnt, ephrin, hedgehog, and STAT genes, as well as resultant deficits in the retinoic acid signaling pathways.[21] Similarly, nonsyndromic craniosynostosis was found to be associated with a nonmendelian inheritance pattern but also frequently involves mutations in the Wnt, BMP, and Ras/ERK pathways.[20] Another study by Wilkie and colleagues[22] used targeted molecular genetics and cytogenetic testing for 326 children born between 1993 and 2002 who required craniosynostosis repair, and they discovered that a genetic diagnosis was achievable in 21% of cases and was associated with an increased risk of complications. Therefore, genetic work-ups are integral to the management of patients with craniosynostosis and contribute to both risk assessment and overall prognosis.[8,20,22]

## OROFACIAL FEATURES OF COMMON CRANIOSYNOSTOSIS SYNDROMES

There are pathognomonic features found in the 4 most common craniosynostosis syndromes (Muenke, Crouzon, Pfieffer, and Apert).[10,16–19] Muenke syndrome is an autosomal dominant disorder with an estimated incidence of 1 in 30,000 live births.[3,16,22] It is characterized by either unicoronal or bicoronal synostosis.[16] Patients with Muenke syndrome present with macrocephaly, midface hypoplasia, and developmental delay. Occlusal findings are typical of a class III skeletal pattern, including anterior crossbite, class III molar and canine relationship, and a concave profile.

Crouzon syndrome is an autosomal dominant disorder and is estimated to affect 1 in 25,000 live births.[9,17] Patients with Crouzon syndrome present most commonly with bicoronal synostosis, brachycephaly, shallow orbits with ocular proptosis, hypertelorism, midface hypoplasia, and relative mandibular prognathism.[17] Those with Crouzon syndrome show maxillary deficiency in the vertical, transverse, and sagittal dimensions and typically present with anterior open bite, posterior and anterior crossbites, and severe crowding of the maxillary arch.[17,23,24] Frequently, teeth become impacted (usually canines) or erupt labially/palatally because of severe teeth-to-arch size discrepancies. Those with severe midface hypoplasia may have lip incompetence and localized areas of gingival inflammation.

Although most cases of Apert syndrome are sporadic, an autosomal dominant inheritance pattern has been reported.[18] It affects 1 in 100,000 live births.[9,18] It is similar in presentation to Crouzon syndrome but with more severe midface hypoplasia, and with syndactyly of the fingers and toes. Apert syndrome is characterized by 1-year to 2-year delay in dental development as well as delayed eruption of the teeth, crowding of upper teeth, and skeletal discrepancy between the maxilla and mandible.[25] Boulet and colleagues[3] estimate that 40% of patients with syndromic craniosynostosis have Apert syndrome. Those with Apert syndrome present with hypoplastic maxillary growth and airway restriction resulting in mouth breathing and anterior open bites, and therefore orthodontic intervention during growth could play a pivotal role in reducing the impact of the developing dentofacial deformity.[26] A distinctive feature in those with Apert syndrome is the presence of bulbous lateral palatal swellings that give the appearance of a pseudocleft. Retention of food and inflammation of surrounding tissues are common findings in such cases.[25–28] Presence of syndactyly frequently precludes patients from following adequate oral hygiene protocols, resulting in poor oral hygiene, increased risk of caries, and gingivitis.[25–28]

Pfeiffer syndrome is autosomal dominant and occurs in 1 in 100,000 live births.[19,29] Pfeiffer syndrome is divided in to 3 subtypes: type I Pfieffer syndrome is the classic manifestation presenting with midface hypoplasia, brachydactyly, and variable syndactyly.[19,29] Cloverleaf skull along with Pfeiffer hands/feet and ankyloses of elbows is the typical presentation of type II. Type III presents with all the features of type II with the exception of Cloverleaf skull. Patients with type III also present with severe ocular proptosis, very short anterior cranial base, and visceral malformations.[19,29]

## SURGICAL MANAGEMENT DURING EARLY YEARS

Management of patients with craniosynostosis requires multidisciplinary care teams that include a pediatric neurologist, geneticist, plastic surgeon, oral and maxillofacial surgeon, neurosurgeon, pediatric dentist, and other specialists ideally in a tertiary health care center. During the first few years of life, treatment mainly involves surgical intervention to relieve the fused sutures. The goal is to reduce the risk of increased ICP, improve the head shape, and allow normal brain development.[4,8–12] Commonly performed surgical procedures include fronto-orbital advancement, open cranial vault remodeling, extended strip craniectomy, endoscopic strip craniectomy, spring-assisted cranial expansion, and cranial vault distraction. Although techniques for initial cranial vault expansion and reshaping depend on the location and extent of the deformity, variability in surgical practice patterns and surgeon experience has been reported in a recent national survey of craniofacial surgeons in the United States.[11] Complication rates also vary widely across different centers, ranging from 10% to 39%.[30–35]

## COMBINED ORTHODONTIC AND SURGICAL TREATMENT PROTOCOLS AND TIMING WITH CASE EXAMPLES

Dentists play a pivotal role in the continuum of care for patients with craniosynostosis.[36] It is recommended that oral health providers conduct a clinical examination following the early surgical management of craniosynostosis. Photographs, diagnostic models, and imaging records should be obtained at periodic intervals to assess growth and eruption of teeth. **Table 1** summarizes the key dental interventions at different time periods.

### Midface Advancement

Much controversy exists on the timing of midface advancement. Some craniofacial teams recommend doing the midface advancement (either with distraction or standard Le Fort III osteotomy procedures) early in life to ameliorate sleep apnea and as an alternative to tracheostomy.[36] Indications for early midface advancement (before growth of midface is complete) include obstructive sleep apnea, globe protection, and psychosocial reasons. It is generally recommended that midface advancement be accomplished between 7 and 12 years of age so as to minimize repeat surgical procedures. There will not be much forward growth of the midface following the surgical

**Table 1**
**Key dental interventions**

| Age (y) | Dentition Stage | Interventions | Providers Involved |
|---------|-----------------|---------------|--------------------|
| <1 | Primary dentition | Establish dental home | Pediatric dentist |
| 1–6 | Primary dentition | • Periodic oral examinations<br>• Assessments for growth<br>• Supervised oral hygiene practices/aids<br>• Maxillary expansion when possible to facilitate incisor and molar eruption | Pediatric dentist, orthodontist, and oral and maxillofacial surgeon |
| 7–12 | Mixed dentition | • Oral hygiene assessments and prophylaxis as needed<br>• Phase I orthodontic treatment (eg, maxillary expansion to correct posterior crossbites, limited maxillary arch orthodontic treatment to correct anterior crossbites, limited orthodontic treatment to facilitate eruption of permanent dentition, and reverse-pull headgear treatment)<br>• Sequential extractions of primary teeth to facilitate eruption of permanent teeth<br>• Midface advancement (as needed) | Pediatric dentist, periodontist, orthodontist, and oral and maxillofacial surgeon |
| 13–21 | Permanent dentition | • Periodic oral examinations, hygiene assessments, and prophylaxis<br>• Comprehensive phase of orthodontic treatment with or without orthognathic surgery (depending on degree of skeletal imbalance)<br>• Restorative treatment (eg, implants, crowns, veneers) following completion of comprehensive phase of orthodontic treatment | Orthodontist, oral and maxillofacial surgeon, periodontist, and prosthodontist |
| >21 | Permanent dentition | • Retention checks<br>• Periodic observations to assess long-term stability of surgical corrections<br>• Periodic oral hygiene visits | Orthodontist, oral and maxillofacial surgeon, and periodontist |

procedure and hence these procedures should be done close to when growth is complete.[24,37]

## Case example for Midface Advancement Using Distraction

Patients with syndromic craniosynostosis present with severe midface hypoplasia. Many have sleep apnea as a result of retropalatal airway collapse.[38,39] When obstructive sleep apnea is present and is not adequately treated with nonoperative maneuvers and tonsillectomy/adenoidectomy, an early midface advancement is recommended. This article presents the case of a female patient, 7 years 2 months old, with Pfeiffer syndrome (type 1) who presented with severe obstructive sleep apnea, concave profile, mixed dentition stage, constricted maxillary arch, posterior and anterior crossbites, anterior open bite, and class III molar relationship (**Figs. 1–3**).

The treatment objectives at this time were to correct the obstructive sleep apnea and improve the profile. To accomplish these objectives, the patient had a midface advancement using distraction osteogenesis. Le Fort III osteotomies were completed and a rigid external distraction device was applied with fixation to the midface using bone-anchored miniplates (**Fig. 4**). At the time of surgery, 3 mm of distraction was performed. Thereafter, 1 mm of distraction per day was done for a total of 10 days followed by 0.5 mm of distraction per day for 2 days. The amount of distraction to be done was decided by airway improvement and polysomnography. A reverse-pull headgear was used for retention for 1 year

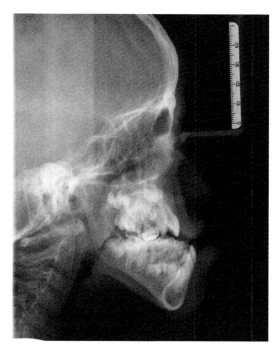

**Fig. 1.** Lateral cephalometric radiograph (at time of presentation).

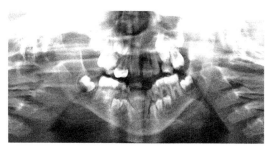

**Fig. 2.** Panoramic radiograph (at time of initial presentation).

following distraction. The 1-year postdistraction intraoral pictures and lateral cephalometric radiograph are presented in **Figs. 5** and **6** respectively.

### Phase I Orthodontic Treatment

Phase I orthodontic treatment usually involves maxillary expansion. Patients with syndromic craniosynostosis present with severely constricted maxillary arches that manifest as posterior crossbites and incompatible arch forms. It is critical that the maxillary arch form be established early, including correction of posterior crossbites to minimize facial asymmetry and eliminate traumatic occlusion. Depending on the severity of maxillary arch constriction, several rounds of expansion may be required. It is best to use a 4-banded expansion appliance if adequate anterior (primary first molars or primary canines) and posterior abutments (permanent first molars) are present, and overexpansion (by about 30%) should be achieved to account for expected relapse. The expansion appliance (usually hyrax, W arch, or quad helix) should be in place for at least 3 months and a fixed transpalatal arch with mesial extension arms should be placed at the time of device removal. Hawley appliances (with acrylic covering of the palate) can also be used, but these need to be periodically adjusted as the primary teeth exfoliate and permanent teeth emerge. It is most efficient to correct transverse maxillary deficiency during the mixed dentition phase when the circum-maxillary and palatal sutures are patent. As the patient ages, the palatal suture becomes fused and there is a considerable amount of resistance from the circum-maxillary sutures to maxillary expansion. In such situations, a surgically assisted maxillary expansion may be required.

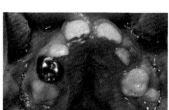
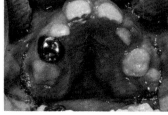

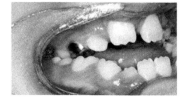
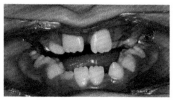
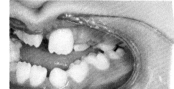

**Fig. 3.** Intraoral views (at time of initial presentation).

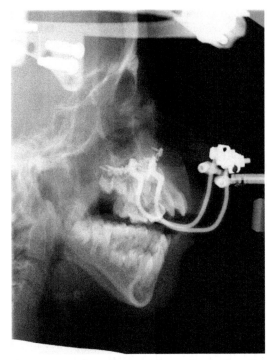

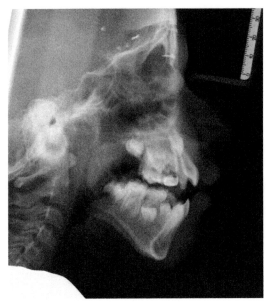

Fig. 6. Lateral cephalometric radiograph 1 year postdistraction.

Fig. 4. Lateral cephalometric radiograph after completion of midfacial distraction.

Occasionally, a limited phase of orthodontic treatment is recommended in the maxillary arch to align and level the arch in preparation for a maxillary advancement operation. Limited orthodontic treatment is also recommended to facilitate eruption of permanent teeth into an ideal position in the arch and for treating impacted teeth. It is best that this phase of treatment not be beyond 6 to 9 months to prevent patient burnout.

## Case example for Surgically Assisted Maxillary Expansion and Limited Orthodontic Treatment

A 16-year-old male patient presented with severe constriction of the maxillary arch, anterior open bite, and severe crowding of both maxillary and mandibular arches (**Fig. 7**). Treatment objectives were to relieve the crowding in both arches, expand the maxillary arch and make it compatible with the mandibular arch, and align/level both arches with a limited phase of orthodontic treatment. A surgically assisted maxillary expansion was done along with extractions of maxillary and mandibular permanent canines, which had

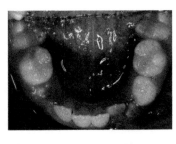
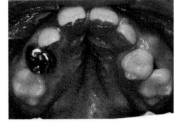
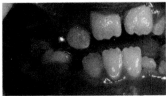
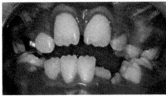
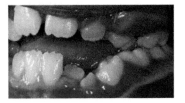

Fig. 5. Intraoral views 1 year postdistraction.

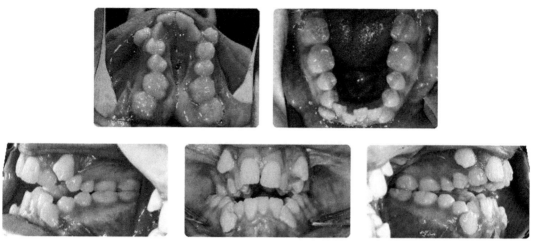

**Fig. 7.** Initial presentation.

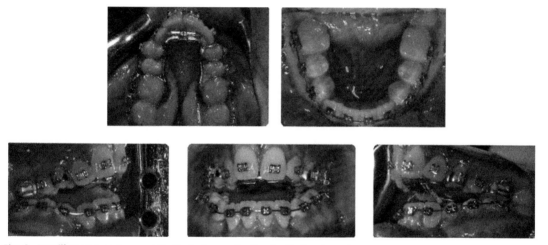

**Fig. 8.** Maxillary expansion and limited phase of orthodontic treatment.

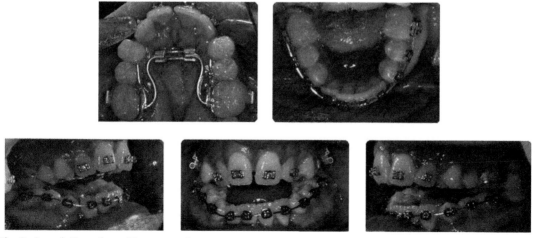

**Fig. 9.** Completion of maxillary expansion.

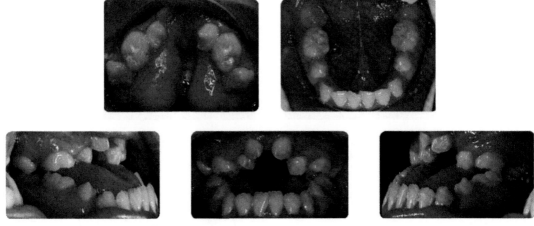

Fig. 10. Intraoral views at initial presentation.

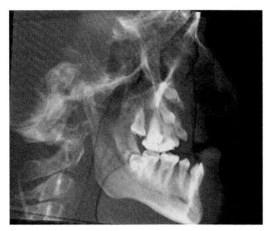

Fig. 11. Lateral cephalometric radiograph at initial presentation.

erupted labially because of severe teeth material/arch length discrepancy. Considering the severely constricted maxillary arch form, 3 rounds of expansions were conducted with a modified maxillary expander (**Figs. 8** and **9**). Comprehensive

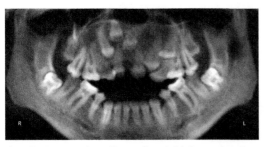

Fig. 12. Panoramic radiograph at initial presentation.

orthodontic treatment in conjunction with orthognathic surgery is planned for the future.

## Comprehensive Orthodontics with Orthognathic Surgery

Most patients with syndromic craniosynostosis present with severe maxillary/mandibular skeletal imbalances and malocclusions that require comprehensive orthodontic treatment in conjunction with orthognathic surgery during the late teen years. Treatment is rendered in 3 stages: presurgical orthodontics, orthognathic surgery, and postsurgical orthodontics. The treatment objectives of these stages are discussed here.

### Presurgical orthodontics
The objectives of this stage are to align and level both maxillary and mandibular arches, obtain compatible arch forms, remove dental compensations (may need extractions of permanent teeth to accomplish this), and resolve crowding/spacing issues.

### Orthognathic surgery
The objectives of this stage are to correct anterior/posterior, transverse, and vertical maxillary/mandibular discrepancies with single jaw or bimaxillary surgery.

### Postsurgical orthodontics
During this stage, the final detailing and settling of occlusion are accomplished.

### Case Example 1 of Comprehensive Orthodontic Treatment with Orthognathic Surgery

A male patient with Apert syndrome presented during the early teen years with a concave profile,

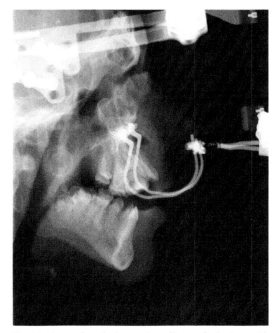

**Fig. 13.** Lateral cephalometric radiograph during midface advancement by distraction.

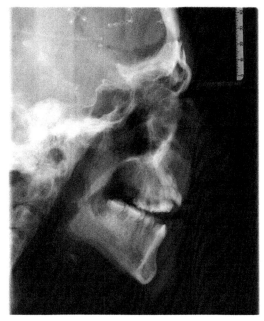

**Fig. 14.** Lateral cephalometric radiograph 1 year postdistraction.

multiple missing teeth in the maxillary arch, anterior open bite, and anterior crossbite (**Figs. 10–12**). Considering the severity of the anterior/posterior imbalance between the maxillary and mandibular arches and severe midface hypoplasia, the treatment was planned in 2 phases. During the initial phase, the patient had midface distraction (**Figs. 13–15**). During the late teen years, the patient underwent a comprehensive phase of orthodontic treatment along with orthognathic surgery (**Figs. 16–18**).

## Case Example 2 of Comprehensive Orthodontic Treatment with Orthognathic Surgery

A male patient with a diagnosis of Apert syndrome presented during the early mixed dentition stage with an impacted maxillary left central incisor (**Fig. 19**). A limited phase of orthodontic treatment was done with the objective of facilitating eruption of the impacted tooth into the arch (**Figs. 20 and 21**). Space was created for the impacted tooth, a surgical exposure was

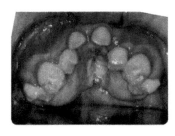
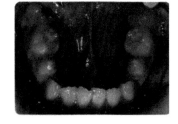
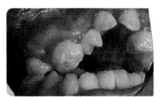
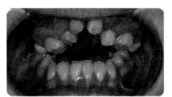
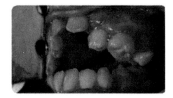

**Fig. 15.** Intraoral views 1 year postdistraction.

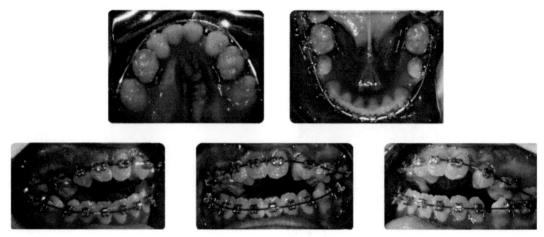

**Fig. 16.** Intraoral views during comprehensive phase of orthodontic treatment (3 years postdistraction).

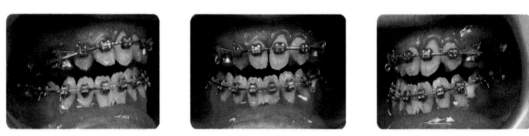

**Fig. 17.** Intraoral views before orthognathic surgery.

done, and orthodontic traction was placed to erupt the impacted tooth into the arch. At 14 years, the patient presented with concave profile, severe maxillary hypoplasia, anterior openbite, negative overjet, posterior crossbite, and class III malocclusion (**Figs. 22** and **23**). A distraction osteogenesis procedure was done

using Le Fort III osteotomies (**Fig. 24**) at age 14 years. During the late teen years, the patient had a comprehensive phase of orthodontic treatment along with orthognathic surgery (Le Fort I and genioplasty). Following the comprehensive phase of treatment, an excellent outcome was achieved (**Figs. 25–28**).

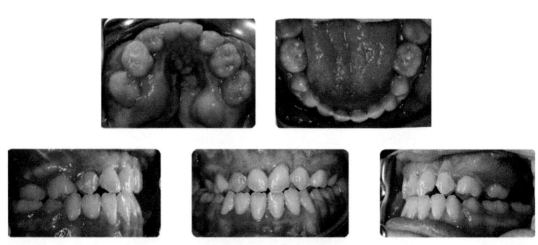

**Fig. 18.** Intraoral views after Le Fort I osteotomy procedure and after debond.

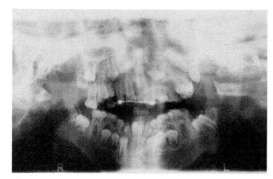

Fig. 19. Panoramic radiograph showing impacted maxillary left central incisor.

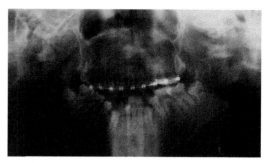

Fig. 21. Panoramic radiograph during limited phase of orthodontic treatment.

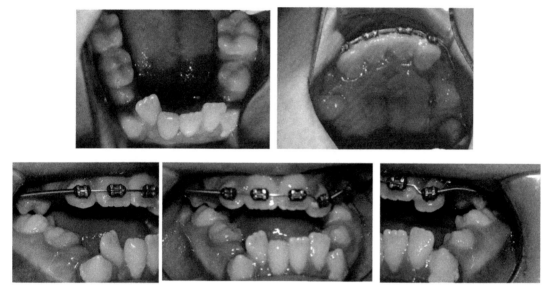

Fig. 20. Intraoral views during limited phase of orthodontic treatment.

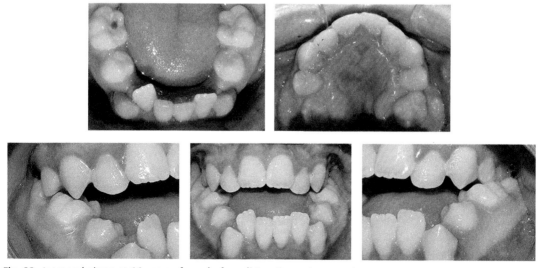

Fig. 22. Intraoral views at 14 years of age before distraction osteogenesis.

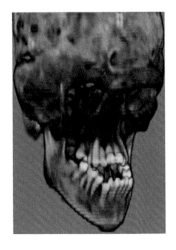
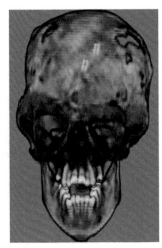
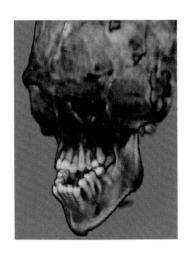

**Fig. 23.** Cone beam computed tomography (CBCT) images before maxillary distraction osteogenesis.

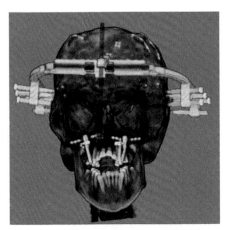
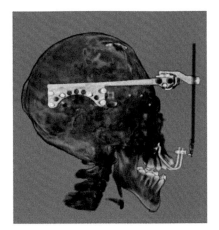

**Fig. 24.** CBCT images during distraction osteogenesis procedure.

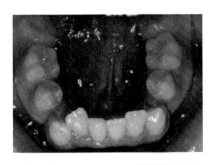
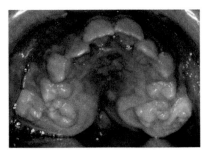

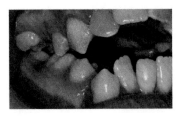
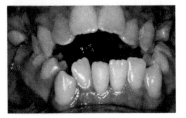
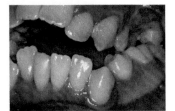

**Fig. 25.** Intraoral views before initiation of comprehensive phase of orthodontic treatment.

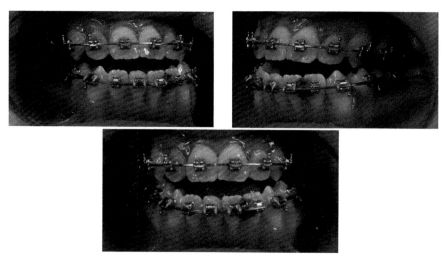

**Fig. 26.** Intraoral views before Le Fort I and genioplasty procedures.

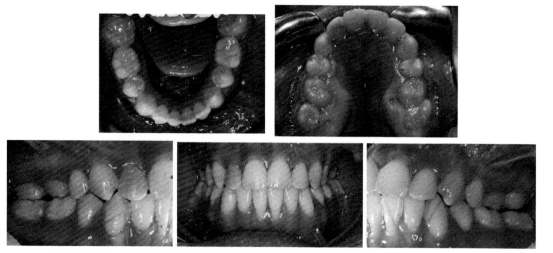

**Fig. 27.** Intraoral views following completion of comprehensive phase of orthodontic treatment.

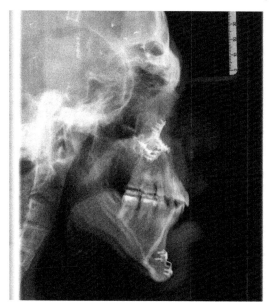

**Fig. 28.** Lateral cephalometric radiograph following completion of comprehensive phase of orthodontic treatment.

## SUMMARY

As shown by the case examples, orthodontic management of syndromic craniosynostosis requires an interdisciplinary approach to treatment, a willingness to understand the limitations inherent (eg, ectopic teeth, impacted teeth, severe maxillary constriction, malformed teeth), and a creative but determined craniofacial orthodontist. Maxillary expansion when done early may reduce but cannot eliminate the occurrence of impaction and the eventual need to extract maxillary permanent teeth, creating the need to design an occlusion providing good function and esthetics. This outcome requires the providers to work together to minimize the amount of intervention (implants, prostheses, phases of orthodontia) needed so as to decrease the overall morbidity of treatment and to reduce the financial and psychological burden on the patient and family.

## DISCLOSURE

The authors have nothing to disclose.

## REFERENCES

1. Singer S, Bower C, Southall P, et al. Craniosynostosis in Western Australia, 1980-1994: a population-based study. Am J Med Genet 1999;83:382–7.
2. Lajeunie E, Le Merrer M, Bonaïti-Pellie C, et al. Genetic study of nonsyndromic coronal craniosynostosis. Am J Med Genet 1995;55:500–4.
3. Boulet SL, Rasmussen SA, Honein MA. A population-based study of craniosynostosis in metropolitan Atlanta, 1989-2003. Am J Med Genet A 2008;146A: 984–91.
4. Renier D, Lajeunie E, Arnaud E, et al. Management of craniosynostoses. Childs Nerv Syst 2000;16: 645–58.
5. Persing JA, Jane JA, Shaffrey M. Virchow and the pathogenesis of craniosynostosis: a translation of his original work. Plast Reconstr Surg 1989;83: 738–42.
6. Twigg ST, Wilkie AO. A genetic-pathophysiological framework for craniosynostosis. Am J Hum Genet 2015;97:359–77.
7. Panigrahi I. Craniosynostosis genetics: the mystery unfolds. Indian J Hum Genet 2011;17(2):48–53.
8. Johnson D, Wilkie AO. Craniosynostosis. Eur J Hum Genet 2011;19:369–76.
9. Derderian C, Seaward J. Syndromic craniosynostosis. Semin Plast Surg 2012;26:64–75.
10. Mathijssen IM. Guideline for care of patients with the diagnoses of craniosynostosis: working group on craniosynostosis. J Craniofac Surg 2015;26(6): 1735–807.
11. Alperovich M, Vyas RM, Staffenberg DA. Is Craniosynostosis repair keeping up with the times? Results from the largest national survey on craniosynostosis. J Craniofac Surg 2015;26:1909–13.
12. Nguyen C, Hernandez-Boussard T, Khosla RK, et al. A national study on craniosynostosis surgical repair. Cleft Palate Craniofac J 2013;50(5):555–60.
13. Alderman BW, Fernbach SK, Greene C, et al. Diagnostic practice and the estimated prevalence of craniosynostosis in Colorado. Arch Pediatr Adolesc Med 1997;151:159–64.
14. Shuper A, Merlob P, Grunebaum M, et al. The incidence of isolated craniosynostosis in the newborn infant. Am J Dis Child 1985;139:85–6.
15. Bruce WJ, Chang V, Joyce CJ, et al. Age at time of craniosynostosis repair predicts increased complication rate. Cleft Palate Craniofac J 2018;55(5): 649–54.
16. OMIM # 62849. Muenke Syndrome. OMIM. Available at: https://omim.org/entry/602849. Accessed September 30, 2019.
17. OMIM # 123500. Crouzon Syndrome. OMIM. Available at: https://omim.org/entry/123500. Accessed September 30, 2019.
18. OMIM # 101200. Apert Syndrome. OMIM. Available at: https://omim.org/entry/101200. Accessed September 30, 2019.
19. OMIM # 101600. Pfeiffer Syndrome. OMIM. Available at: https://omim.org/entry/101600. Accessed September 30, 2019.
20. Timberlake AT, Persing JA. Genetics of nonsyndromic craniosynostosis. Plast Reconstr Surg 2018;141(6):1508–16.
21. Twigg SRF, Vorgia E, Mcgowan SJ, et al. Reduced dosage of ERF causes complex craniosynostosis in humans and mice and links ERK1/2 signaling to regulation of osteogenesis. Nat Genet 2013;405: 308–13.
22. Wilkie AO, Byren JC, Hurst JA, et al. Prevalence and complications of single-gene and chromosomal disorders in craniosynostosis. Pediatrics 2010;126(2): e391–400.
23. Kreiborg S. Crouzon Syndrome. A clinical and roentgencephalometric study. Scand J Plast Reconstr Surg Suppl 1981;18:1–198.
24. Kreiborg S, Aduss H. Pre- and postsurgical facial growth in patients with Crouzon's and Apert's syndromes. Cleft Palate J 1986;23(Suppl 1):78–90.
25. Kaloust S, Ishii K, Vargervik K. Dental development in Apert syndrome. Cleft Palate Craniofac J 1997; 34:117–21.
26. Letra A, the Almeida AL, Kaizer R, et al. Intraoral features of Apert's syndrome. Oral Surg Oral Med Oral Pathol Oral Radiol Endod 2007;103:e38–41.
27. Ferraro NF. Dental, orthodontic, and oral/maxillofacial evaluation and treatment in Apert syndrome. Clin Plast Surg 1991;18(2):291–307.
28. Paravatty RP, Ahsan A, Sebastian BT, et al. Apert syndrome: a case report with discussion of craniofacial features. Quintessence Int 1999;30(6):423–6.
29. National Organization of Rare Disorders. Pfeiffer syndrome. Available at: https://rarediseases.org/rare-diseases/pfeiffer-syndrome/. Accessed September 30, 2019.
30. Lee HQ, Hutson JM, Wray AC, et al. Analysis of morbidity and mortality in surgical management of craniosynostosis. J Craniofac Surg 2012;23:1256–61.
31. Esparza J, Hinojosa J, García-Recuero I, et al. Surgical treatment of isolated and syndromic craniosynostosis. Results and complications in 283 consecutive cases. Neurocirugia (Astur) 2008;19: 509–29.
32. Esparza J, Hinojosa J. Complications in the surgical treatment of craniosynostosis and craniofacial syndromes: Apropos of 306 transcranial procedures. Childs Nerv Syst 2008;24:1421–30.
33. Jeong JH, Song JY, Kwon GY, et al. The results and complications of cranial bone reconstruction in

patients with craniosynostosis. J Craniofac Surg 2013;24:1162–7.

34. Pearson GD, Havlik RJ, Eppley B, et al. Craniosynostosis: a single institution's outcome assessment from surgical reconstruction. J Craniofac Surg 2008;19:65–71.

35. Chattha A, Bucknor A, Curiel DA, et al. Treatment of craniosynostosis: the impact of hospital surgical volume on cost, resource utilization, and outcomes. J Craniofac Surg 2018;29(5):1233–6.

36. Vargervik K, Rubin MS, Grayson BH, et al. Parameters of care for craniosynostosis: dental and orthodontic perspectives. Am J Orthod Dentofacial Orthop 2012;141(4 Suppl):S68–73.

37. Shetye PR, Kapadia H, Grayson BH, et al. A 10-year study of skeletal stability and growth of the midface following Le Fort III advancement in syndromic craniosynostosis. Plast Reconstr Surg 2010;126(3): 973–81.

38. Inverso G, Brustowicz KA, Katz E, et al. The prevalence of obstructive sleep apnea in symptomatic patients with syndromic craniosynostosis. Int J Oral Maxillofac Surg 2016;45(2):167–9.

39. Resnick CM, Middleton JK, Calabrese CE, et al. Retropalatal cross-sectional area is predictive of obstructive sleep apnea in patients with syndromic craniosynostosis. Cleft Palate Craniofac J 2019. https://doi.org/10.1177/1055665619882571.

# Orthodontic Considerations for Cleft Orthognathic Surgery

Stephen Yen, DMD, PhD[a],*, Jeffrey Hammoudeh, DDS, MD[b],
Sean P. Edwards, DDS, MD[c], Mark Urata, DDS, MD[d]

## KEYWORDS

- Cleft lip and palate • Class III malocclusion • Surgical and orthodontic treatment
- Cleft orthognathic surgery

## KEY POINTS

- Preparation and planning for orthognathic surgery in late adolescence depends on the complexity of unresolved problems with which the patient presents.
- Different strategies are presented to address these unresolved problems in the adult patient with cleft lip and palate.
- Different surgical and orthodontic treatments are presented to correct the class III malocclusion in patients with cleft lip and palate in ranges that are analogous to the envelope of discrepancy.
- For complex cases, the principles of achievability, stability, and esthetics should guide the decision-making process for planning the preparation for orthognathic surgery.

Planning orthognathic surgery for the patient with cleft lip and palate can be challenging. By the time a patient with cleft lip and palate has completed adolescent growth and is ready for orthognathic surgery, the patient will present with a problem list that is based on the severity of the original cleft defect and the types of treatment that were used to address the primary lip and palate repairs, nasal revision, alveolar bone grafting, velopharyngeal insufficiency, and palatal fistulas. With staged and coordinated team care,[1] it is hoped the patient will not need orthognathic surgery or will have a class III malocclusion that is easily managed with a LeFort 1 surgery. However, in large urban hospitals like Children's Hospital Los Angeles or the Los Angeles County/University of Southern California (USC) Hospital, many of the authors' patients are transfer patients from other hospitals or had primary surgeries done elsewhere, sometimes in other parts of the world, and present with challenging malocclusions. Some patients did not receive earlier care or missed optimal timing for the different types of treatment. During the author's initial examination, questions to ascertain the treatment history are not meant to assign blame as to how the patient got to this point; rather, they are designed to find out what worked or did not work for the patient and to use the information to develop strategies to solve the combination of problems with which they presented. For example, the authors' first rigid external distraction (RED) maxillary distraction case was for an adult patient with cleft lip and palate and maxillary hypoplasia with a 14-mm anterior cross-bite (**Fig. 1**). He was unsuccessfully treated with a LeFort I maxillary

[a] Division of Dentistry, Children's Hospital Los Angeles, 4650 Sunset Blvd, MS 116, Los Angeles, CA 90027, USA;
[b] Division of Oral and Maxillofacial Surgery, Department of Plastic and Reconstructive Surgery, Children's Hospital Los Angeles, MS 96, CA 90275, USA; [c] University of Michigan, Mott Children's Hospital, Floor 3, Reception B, 1540 E Hospital Dr, SPC 4219, Ann Arbor, MI 48109-4219, USA; [d] Children's Hospital Los Angeles, MS 96, 4650 Sunset Blvd, Los Angeles, CA 90027, USA
* Corresponding author.
*E-mail address:* syen@usc.edu

Oral Maxillofacial Surg Clin N Am 32 (2020) 249–267
https://doi.org/10.1016/j.coms.2020.01.013

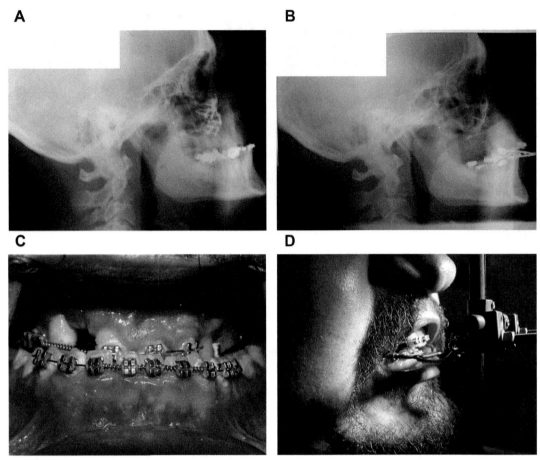

Fig. 1. (*A*) Initial consult: surgical relapse from LeFort I surgery. (*B*) Re-treatment with maxillary distraction using a rigid external distractor. (*C*) Presurgical intraoral view. (*D*) Overcorrection with RED device.

advancement (see **Fig. 1**A), as evidenced by the LeFort I plates still in place but with the 20-mm class III malocclusion. The prior surgeon was an authority on orthognathic surgery, having written on the subject, so the authors assumed the problem was the strategy and not the surgeon or the surgical technique. Rather than repeat the approach, they used a rigid external distractor, RED distractor (KLS Martin, Freiburg, Germany),[2] to distract the maxilla into an overcorrected class II overjet, hoping that gradual lengthening of the maxilla would be more stable than the LeFort I osteotomy (see **Fig. 1**B). In his case, after 5 years, he relapsed to a class I occlusion. One of the challenging questions that craniofacial teams have to face is what should be done when conventional or traditional treatments fail in patients with cleft lip and palate. Should the same approach be repeated or can the approach be changed to improve the outcome? What type of correction is achievable? At the authors' center, when traditional approaches fail to solve a problem, then

alternative approaches are considered to solve difficult problems in cleft care.

## ANOTHER CONSIDERATION IS COST

Seventy percent of the patients seen at Children's Hospital Los Angeles are insured through Medicaid. Similarly, at the Los Angeles County/ USC hospital, most patients have Medicaid and are dependent on government-supported health insurance. At the county hospital, adult patients with cleft lip and palate are too old to be seen at a Children's Hospital or require adult dental services that are not available at Children's Hospital Los Angeles. For the adult patient with cleft lip and palate, there can be a greater number of possible treatment plans because the solution to a malocclusion may be orthodontic, surgical, prosthodontic, or a combination of the three. There may not be a perfect solution because cost, length of treatment, esthetic goals, and stability may come into play in the decision making. Consider

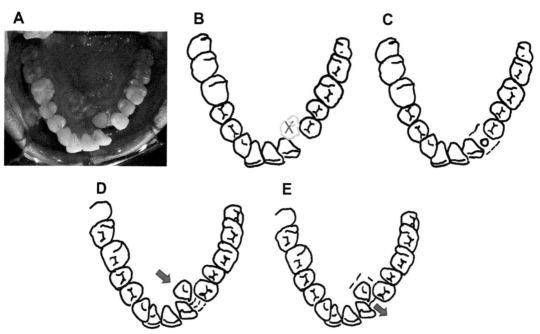

**Fig. 2.** (*A*) Problem of buccal defect due to alveolar cleft and possible solutions. (*B*) Extract tooth, build fixed bridge. (*C*) Graft for dental implant. (*D*) The movement of the tooth into a bone graft. (*E*) The movement of the osteotomized segment to join the archform. (*E*) Segmental osteotomy to move segment containing the tooth into the dental arch with nickel titanium archwires.

**Fig. 2**A, a 41-year old with cleft lip and palate who presents without a 202 One solution is to graft the cleft site and align the tooth (**Fig. 4**D) For this patient, there are multiple treatment options. If the tooth is moved into the dental arch or cleft site, the dental root will leave the alveolar bony housing. One solution is to graft the cleft site and align the tooth. Another solution is to apply braces, create a box osteotomy around the canine dental root, and distract the bony segment into the archform with nickel titanium archwires (**Fig. 2**E). This treatment plan would allow the patient to use her own teeth and align her crowded anterior teeth but will lengthen her treatment time. Given that the prognosis of the tooth is already questionable because of periodontal disease, another solution could be to extract the canine and fabricate a bridge and veneers or graft the alveolar cleft and place a dental implant (**Fig. 2**C). To offer options like orthognathic surgery, dental implants, orthodontics, prosthodontics, and periodontics implies that a comprehensive set of services are available and affordable to the craniofacial team and patient, which is not always the case for state-supported patient care. For this patient, it will be important to discuss the treatment options, the possible outcomes, length of treatment, and cost and then weigh what options can be covered under her medical insurance.

## THE TREATMENT CAN BE COMPLEX

Depending on how much treatment a patient with cleft lip and palate received earlier, the orthodontic and surgical treatment plan for an adult or late adolescent patient can be straightforward or challenging. The potential problem list for an adult patient with a cleft lip and palate can be daunting:[3] failed bone grafts, incomplete bone fill from prior bone grafts or gingivoperioplasty, large cleft defects that comprise missing bone, teeth, and soft tissue, exposed roots of permanent teeth along the edge of the cleft, large palatal fistula, poor speech, dental anomalies such as hypodontia, microdontia, transposition, large class III malocclusions, transverse width deficiencies, overerupted lower incisors due to lack of opposing teeth, canting of the occlusal plane, decreased vertical dentoalveolar development of the maxillary teeth and inadequate display of incisors, ectopic eruption and dental crowding within cleft segments, deviated maxillary dental midlines, and cleft segments that are not on the same occlusal plane or are canted vertically into "a keeled position." Fortunately, the toolbox for craniofacial orthodontics and surgery is extensive and borrows from many different reconstructive strategies. The purpose of this article is to illustrate some strategies for complex cleft-related problems.

## REGAINING ARCHFORM AND RESOLVING DENTAL CROWDING

In **Fig. 2**B, a patient presents with a large alveolar cleft and 2 missing teeth. The large cleft defect represents missing tissue: missing bone, missing teeth, and missing soft tissue. With less available bone for dental eruption within each cleft segment, the eruption of permanent teeth may result in ectopic eruption or dental crowding within the ungrafted segments. Ectopic eruption of teeth can occur if there is a net difference between combined tooth size and arch length within a segment due to the missing bone volume within each segment. To treat the dental crowding, the dental archform could be expanded and the cleft site grafted so that the tooth can move into the grafted bone. Alternatively, the ectopic teeth can be extracted and then surgically or orthodontically reposition the segments. However, the patient is already missing two teeth as well as a large amount of alveolar bone. An alternative strategy

can be developed to create additional bone by segmental distraction osteogenesis using temporary anchorage devices (TADs) and segmental bony movement along an archwire. **Fig. 3** illustrates this strategy. After correcting the collapsed position of the lesser segment, segmental osteotomies were created between the canine and premolar so that the osteotomized segment bearing teeth can be distracted along an archwire to constrict the cleft site and dock the segments using TAD and "pull" coil springs. Distraction forces are applied directly to bone and not to the dentition in order to prevent roots from leaving the bone at the leading edge of the distraction segment. The goal was to correct the midline, to create bone for palatal teeth to enter the dental arch, and to make the cleft space smaller for the surgeons to graft.

The next case serves as an illustration of how techniques developed for trauma can be reapplied to craniofacial problems. The authors developed a technique for segmental distraction osteogenesis

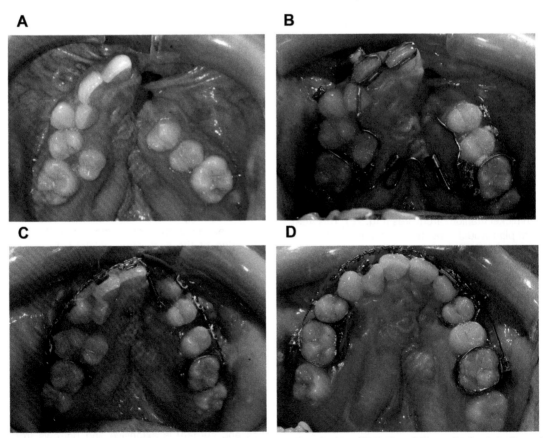

**Fig. 3.** The distorted archform associated with a large cleft defect. (*A*) Collapsed archform of a large unilateral alveolar cleft. (*B*) Correction of the collapsed position. (*C*) Segmental distraction in the greater segment to move the incisor-bearing segment toward the cleft with TADs and coil springs. (*D*) Regaining the archform by moving teeth into the distraction site.

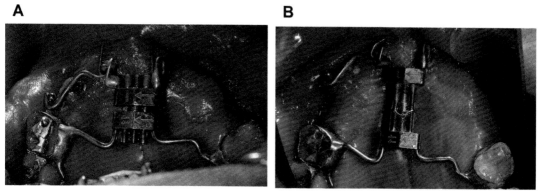

**Fig. 4.** (*A*) Loss of anterior maxilla due to trauma corrected by custom distraction device for AP distraction. (*B*) Lengthening the maxilla by segmental distraction. (*From* Lypka M, Afshar A, Pham D, et al. Implant-supported distraction osteogenesis: a technique to advance the deficient maxilla. J Craniofac Surg. 2009;20(2):526; with permission.)

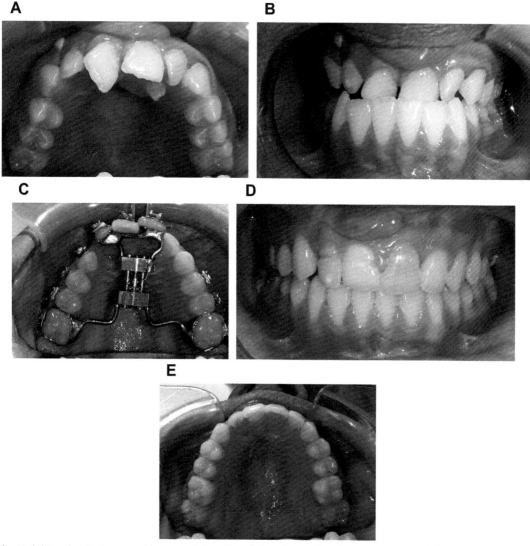

**Fig. 5.** (*A*) Similar strategy used to correct class III and dental crowding in a patient with cleft lip and palate. Presurgical occlusal view. (*B*) Presurgical underbite. (*C*) Distraction device. (*D*) Corrected underbite. (*E*) Postsurgical occlusal view.

to rebuild anterior maxillary bone[4] that was lost because of trauma in a motorcycle accident by using a rapid palatal expansion (RPE) device turned 90° to provide anteroposterior (AP) expansion (**Fig. 4**A, B). Preexisting dental implants were incorporated into the custom distractor so that the anterior segment could be advanced out of an anterior cross-bite in order to consider a fixed bridge rather than a removable prosthesis for the patient. **Fig. 5** illustrates how this same technique was adapted for use with a patient with cleft lip and palate, in order to simultaneously correct a class III malocclusion and maxillary dental crowding. The anterior segmental distraction approach uses gradual lengthening, has a short recovery period, and is well tolerated because the patient adapted to the RPE before surgery. There is no need for intermaxillary fixation, and the patient can resume a normal diet after the mucosa has healed. Similar approaches were reported in the literature this year.[5]

## COGNITIVE DELAY

The patient with syndromic cleft lip and palate and cognitive delay is a special concern because the patient may not be cooperative enough to carry out the treatment. The authors assess the cooperation by taking a panoramic radiograph and dental impressions during their initial data gathering. It is important to assess whether the patient can perform the basic functions of breathing, speech, and eating without difficulty. Because orthodontic treatment relies on patient cooperation, it is helpful to have a motivated patient. Ideally, the patient should be able to explain why they want braces, which would suggest a sense of self-awareness. This level of cooperation and understanding may not be possible for a patient with cognitive delay; therefore, it is important to establish which treatment goals are achievable. For example, serial extractions during mixed dentition can be done under general anesthesia to avoid canine impactions. The treatment should address functional goals and how surgery and limited orthodontics would improve quality of life. Based on prior experience, orthognathic surgery is not recommended to patients who have severe cognitive delay and are in special education because they may react poorly to surgery. For example, when a patient awakens from anesthesia, the patient with cognitive delay may not remember postoperative instructions and may panic if they cannot open their mouths when placed in intermaxillary fixation. Some patients in the past reacted in unexpected ways and attempted to remove the wires or loosen the maxillary segments. Another example is a high

functioning patient with Down's syndrome, who was cooperative throughout treatment, a large prognathic mandible was corrected by mandibular setback surgery. After braces were removed, this patient postured the mandible forward into the presurgical position and functioned by protruding the mandible forward to simulate the presurgical bite. These early experiences have led the authors to avoid surgery for patients with cognitive delay and to offer surgery only if it can lead to a better quality of life for the patient.

## ADDRESSING FAILED BONE GRAFTS

A full-head cone beam computed tomography (CT) and a physical examination are good starting points for evaluating the alveolar cleft site when an alveolar bone graft failed. The data from the cone beam CT will show the size and dimensions of the cleft defect, the anatomic contour of a cleft space in 3 dimensions (3D), and its relationship to dental roots of adjacent teeth. In a recent research thesis,[6] bony voids in bone grafts were associated with bone grafts placed against teeth that emerged out of the adjacent bone into the cleft space. Bone can graft to bone but not to cementum or enamel. The cone beam CT can show crowns of supernumerary teeth or exposed dental roots in the cleft site that might need extracting in order to avoid grafting bone against dental enamel or cementum. Early bone grafting may be the solution for preventing the emergence of incisor roots and crowns into the cleft site.[7,8] If the expanded position is too large, then a critical size defect is created, which may be difficult to graft. In order to give the surgeons the best chance to graft the cleft space with tension-free flaps, the segments are brought closer together using the nasoalveolar molding principle of moving the segments into a docking position before grafting. TADs are placed in the segments that need constriction in order to avoid placing elastic force on teeth adjacent to the cleft site that could potentially move dental roots out of bone. Passive archwires and expansion devices are used for stabilizing cleft segments for the bone graft; whenever the cleft adjacent teeth occlude against the lower dentition, a posterior bite plate or surgical splint is used to separate the incisors and protect the graft site from traumatic occlusion.

If there is partial bone fill from the bone graft or gingivoperioplasty, then the cone beam CT can show whether a regraft should be attempted and whether adjacent teeth in the cleft site should be removed. Whenever possible, primary teeth or supernumerary teeth can be moved into new bone grafts to help maintain bone height and

A

B

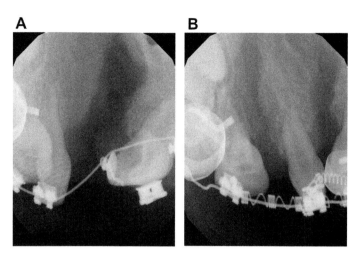

**Fig. 6.** (*A*) Large residual cleft after first bone graft. The primary canine is part of the lesser segment. (*B*) Segmental distraction with a bony segment containing the primary canine was used to produce bone in the cleft site before grafting the docked segments.

volume. In some unusually large alveolar clefts,[9,10] the authors will use segmental distraction, TADs, and archwires to distract a bony segment containing a tooth across the cleft space and dock with the opposite cleft segment before grafting (**Figs. 6** and **7**). For the adult patient who has not had a secondary bone graft, the craniofacial team will need to decide whether to stage the bone graft before the orthognathic surgery or whether to simultaneously graft the cleft segments while advancing the maxilla during the LeFort I surgery.

## USING ECTOPIC PALATAL TEETH

It can be useful to save ectopic palatal teeth even if the teeth are microdonts because these teeth can be used to preserve graft height, transport bone

A          B          C

D          E

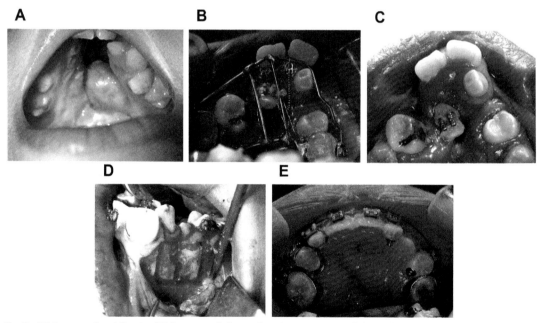

**Fig. 7.** (*A*) Large palatal fistula. (*B*) Segmental distraction that transported the palatal tooth across the fistula. (*C*) Collapsed archform and closure of fistula after bony transport. (*D*) Corticotomies to assist wire expansion. (*E*) Restored archform and fistula closure. (*Adapted from* Yen SL, Yamashita DD, Kim TH, et al. Closure of an unusually large palatal fistula in a cleft patient by bony transport and corticotomy-assisted expansion. J Oral Maxillofac Surg. 2003;61(11):1347; with permission; and Yen SL, Yamashita DD, Gross J, et al. Combining orthodontic tooth movement with distraction osteogenesis to close cleft spaces and improve maxillary arch form in cleft lip and palate patients. Am J Orthod Dentofacial Orthop. 2005;127(2):2228; with permission.)

through a cleft site (**Fig. 6**), transport bone through a large palatal defect, and support a resin crown or Maryland bridge. During growth, if the microdont is moved into a bone graft in the position of a missing lateral incisor, the tooth will maintain the height of the bone graft during the interim period between the placement of the graft and the placement of a dental implant. Also, in cases of missing lateral incisors, a microdont can provide stability as a third point of contact for a Maryland bridge replacement of a lateral incisor. The Maryland bridge wings are bonded to the flanking central incisor and canine, but it is also bonded to the occlusal surface of the microdont. The microdont will resist torquing forces that normally cause Maryland bridges to come loose. In a case with an unusually large palatal fistula, the authors reported how a palatal tooth was used to close the anterior palatal fistula (see **Fig. 7**).[11] A palatal positioned primary tooth in a patient who had a 21-mm anterior palatal fistula was used to distract a plate of bone across the anterior palatal fistula and create additional soft tissue for palatal closure. The patient had 3 failed tongue flaps from multiple reputable craniofacial centers, so the authors changed the strategy to a custom palatal distraction device that eventually closed the palatal defect.[11] The palatal fistula was closed by a combination of palatal segmental distraction and collapsing the archform. Buccal corticotomies and wire expansion were used to regain the archform without enlarging the fistula. In animal experiments, the authors found that any segment smaller than 1 cm × 1 cm would fracture if a predrilled screw was placed in the bony plate. The palatal tooth became the screw for

moving the tooth, bone, and soft tissue across the palatal defect, thereby reducing the defect so that it could be closed.

A more common problem is the palatal-displaced canine, as seen in **Fig. 2**A. If the canine erupted palatally, after bone grafting, the cortical alveolar bone may be deficient on the buccal side for tooth movement into the archform. There is a buccal depression in the alveolar bone that the palatal canine has to move into. Because of the thin buccal bone, the dental roots may move out of bone if they are moved into the dental arch. In these situations, a box osteotomy can be made around the canine, and the tooth-bearing segment can be brought into the archform by a custom distractor,[12] as illustrated in **Fig. 8**A, or by nickel titanium wires that can move the box segment into the archform. To minimize the risk of losing the segment containing the canine, a passive archwire is preinserted to stabilize the segment during the 2-day latency period. This archwire is replaced with an active nickel titanium archwire. A rectangular or square nickel titanium archwire is placed a week later to add torque to the segmental position.

## ALIGNING A MUTILATED DENTITION

Because 60% to 70% of patients with cleft lip and palate have a missing lateral incisor [13] and the remaining 30% may have some form of dental anomaly affecting the mesiodistal dimensions of the dental arch, severe Bolton discrepancies are expected in the patient with cleft lip and palate. The goal of intercuspation may be achievable for

**A**

**B**

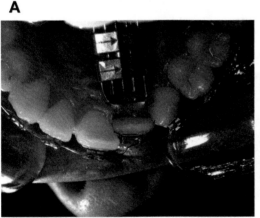
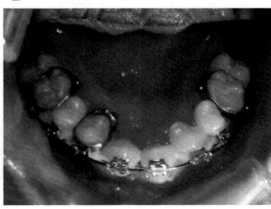

**Fig. 8.** (*A*) Single tooth distractor to move osteotomized segment containing tooth into the archform. (*B*) The problem of the missing premaxilla: collapsing the lateral segments allows the lateral segments to dock before bone grafting. This strategy places 2 canines at the maxillary midline. (*From* Yen SL, Yamashita DD, Gross J, et al. Combining orthodontic tooth movement with distraction osteogenesis to close cleft spaces and improve maxillary arch form in cleft lip and palate patients. Am J Orthod Dentofacial Orthop. 2005;127(2):2228; with permission.)

1 segment but not the other because the maxillary arch might have a combination of missing teeth, transposition, a posterior tooth in the curved portion of the dental archform, and teeth of different sizes. This mutilated maxillary dentition must occlude against a normal dentition in the mandibular arch. For such cases, a Kesling wax setup or digital orthodontic software, like Invisalign, Orthoanalyzer, or Nemotec, can help plan how to arrange the spacing between teeth to optimize the intercuspation. Although the technology exists for trying out different orthodontic setups, final outcomes are hard to foresee at an early age or before surgery because surgical outcomes are less predictable in the patient with cleft lip and palate. The authors tend to use a wait-and-see approach when the patient is in their adolescent growth spurt. If new problems arise, then additional surgeries may be needed. When the authors see the patient as an adult or late adolescent with residual problems, some treatments may have relapsed, or mandibular growth may have occurred requiring retreatment and reoperation. In practice, a progress model taken after the first rectangular wire is placed is useful to assess the intercuspation, overall occlusion, and orthodontic setup. Errors in leveling and bracket height positions should be addressed at this time as well as second molar positioning. In an extremely short maxilla, the posterior teeth may be forced to tip buccally, especially in a relative class III crossbite, and the incisors may be in a proclined position despite extractions to decompensate their position. To correct buccal root torque as seen from a posterior view of the models, nitinol expanders that can be programmed by electric current[14] are useful for torquing the molar roots to correct the buccal tipping to its correct upright position. TADs can also help in correcting molar root torque.

In cases with a missing premaxilla and large cleft defects, the cleft segments may be missing a lateral and central incisor as well as premolars. The juxtaposition of these shortened segments near the midline could place a premolar or molar close to the midline (**Fig. 8**B). The segments are collapsed to the midline in order to narrow the cleft space that needs to be grafted. The authors tend to use expanders that work in the opposite direction from an expanded to a collapsed screw position. Alternatively, the authors can use TADs, as seen in **Fig. 3**. Eventually, curved stainless steel rectangular wires are needed to prepare these patients for orthognathic surgery; however, a rectangular wire cannot insert into a linear molar tube that is near the center of a curve without distortion, making the archform more V shaped than U shaped. Different brackets and final wires may be needed to address this unusual problem, which is a departure from conventional surgical preparation.

## CORRECTING MIDLINES

If the midline is to be corrected with asymmetric extraction and orthodontic tooth movement, then the bone graft must be assessed to determine whether the alveolar bone is adequate for orthodontic tooth movement. If the graft has an hourglass shape that is too narrow in the middle of the alveolar ridge for orthodontic tooth movement, then the Zachrisson technique[15] of alternating 1 month of tooth movement using light spring force with 1 month of spring removal and wire ligation can be used. The pause in tooth movement allows the bone formation to catch up to the leading edge of the bone. This technique was developed to move teeth into atrophic alveolar ridges, which are what an edentulous bone graft may become. If surgery is to be used to correct a midline, then it is important to assess maxillary yaw. In large cleft defects, the collapsed archform can swing the midline toward the lesser segment. If there is a 1-cm deviation of the maxillary midline, then during the maxillary advancement, 1 side will have an additional 1 cm of advancement to correct the midline. If the combined lengthening of class III correction and yaw correction is very large, then the surgery may become less stable. A compromise that is less esthetic but more stable is AP class III correction without rotating the maxilla so that the lateral incisor is left in the central incisor position and reshaped into a central incisor. This strategy was adopted once after a LeFort I surgery that corrected both the class III malocclusion and midline relapsed. The benefits and risks of optimal versus achievable goals were reassessed during the planning for the second surgery. Finally, if the midline needs to be corrected at the end of orthognathic surgery, maxillary distraction, or protraction, it is possible to move the midline the distance of 1 incisor using asymmetric TADs and springs, placed in the canine region, and one in the opposite molar region (**Fig. 9**). Unfortunately, treatment time will be extended at least 1 year for this correction.

## LEVELING THE OCCLUSAL PLANE AND MAINTAINING THE PERIODONTIUM

Conventional orthodontic leveling techniques are normally used to level the maxillary dentition in the noncleft patient. However, the patient with cleft lip and palate may have cleft segments that have

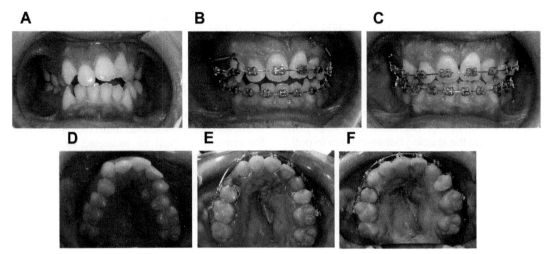

**Fig. 9.** Midline correction with TADs and orthodontics. (*A*) Frontal view of midline to the left of facial midline. (*B*) Asymmetric TADs used to correct maxillary midline. (*C*) Frontal view of corrected midline. (*D*) Palatal view of displaced midline. (*E*) Palatal view of TADs and springs. (*F*) Palatal view of midline correction.

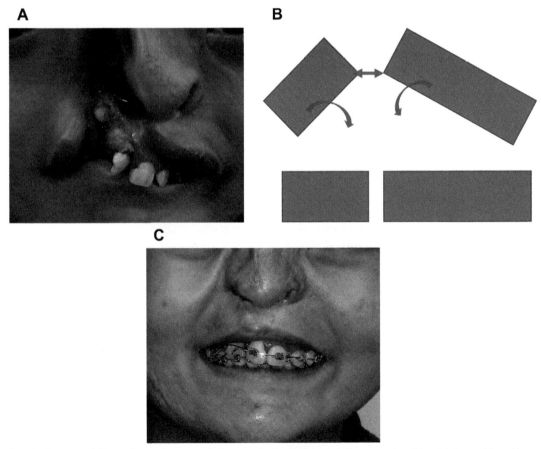

**Fig. 10.** Segmental distraction to lower and align vertically displaced cleft segments without interpositional bone grafts. (*A*) Presurgical facial cleft with "keeled" vertically displaced segments. After segmental osteotomy, a passive archwire keeps segments in original position for callus formation. (*B*) The rotational "downgraft" movement of the osteotomized LeFort 1 segments by elastic nickel titanium archwires (18 x 18 nickel-titanium). A spring is placed between the segments to prevent binding of segments as the segments lower like a drawbridge. (*C*) After leveling of segment and rotation of the central incisors.

collapsed both transversely and vertically into the void of the cleft space. The entire segment may need to be leveled like a drawbridge in cases with large clefts and upward canting of the segments. If vertical elastics are used, then there is the potential for extruding the teeth out of bone and creating periodontal defects (**Fig. 10**A). A strategy for leveling the segments is segmental distraction of cut segments with nickel titanium archwires. Segments can be safely "downgrafted" by segmental distraction and moved into position with osteotomies if a passive stainless steel archwire maintains the osteotomized segment against the host bone during the latency period for vertical segmental distraction. **Fig. 10** is taken from a patient who was brought to the authors' hospital by a surgical mission team in the Philippines. The unrepaired facial cleft had "keeled"[2] or vertically displaced segments that needed to be lowered like a drawbridge without interpositional grafts. The segmental distraction was accomplished using nickel-titanium archwires as the force to mold the segments and to reposition the segment in 3D in order to connect the segment to the dental archform. Initially, a nickel titanium "push" coil spring was placed between osteotomized segments to keep the segments apart and prevent the segments from binding as the segment descends. For these procedures, vestibular incisions were replaced with 2 vertical release incisions so that the buccal mucosa could be moved away from the bone to create a tunnel. The tunnel flap preserved the buccal blood supply. After the outline of the box is cut between and above the dental roots, an osteotome was used to complete the osteotomy. In most cases, a palatal flap can be avoided to protect the palatal blood supply.

The mandibular dentition can present with a different problem in leveling. In a class III malocclusion with underbite, the incisor eruption is left unopposed, and the mandibular anterior teeth can overerupt into a deep underbite. Placement of lingual arches or 2 × 4 archwires during mixed dentition can limit the eruption of the incisors. However, once the incisors have overerupted, then utility arches or Australian 0.016 intrusion arches in tip edge brackets can be used to intrude the anterior dentition during the leveling phase of treatment. Posterior bite blocks and glass ionomer bite turbos can be used to open the bite enough to place brackets on the maxillary anterior teeth. Multiple loop archwires as well as TADs at the mid symphysis can be used to intrude the lower incisors in difficult cases. The juxtaposition of microdonts and transposed teeth may pose a challenge in terms of bracketing of teeth; in these cases, a Kesling setup and bracket height gauge can be useful adjuncts for optimizing the occlusion and marginal ridge height of the posterior teeth.

## ADDRESSING THE TRANSVERSE DIMENSION

It is possible to expand the postgraft maxilla with a rapid palatal expander because it is part of the National Institutes of Health protocol for postgraft maxillary protraction and should be used whenever possible to gain transverse arch width.[16] For patients with bilateral cleft lip and palate and a missing premaxilla, the large intercanine distances were too large to graft; therefore, the segments were collapsed to dock at the midline and were grafted at the midline to make the graft easier to close for the surgeons (see **Fig. 8**B). Afterward, in these extreme cases of narrow maxillae, surgically assisted RPE with an additional cut through the bone graft can create a distraction site to provide additional bone for implants to replace 2 missing central incisors. Unlike vertical alveolar distraction, segmental distraction along an archwire can create an alveolar ridge that is an extension of the host bone with good vertical height for 2 dental implants in the incisor region.

As an example of extreme expansion, **Fig. 11** shows a patient with a lateral cleft and a narrow, distorted maxilla. This patient was corrected in 2004 using telescopic screw expanders, a surgically assisted rapid palatal expansion (SARPE), and TADs to widen the upper maxilla. The screws were placed so that the teeth supporting the RPE would not be pushed out of the alveolar bone during the expansion. The diastema in **Fig. 11**B shows the extent of the expansion. For extreme cases of narrow maxillae in young children, when the RPE screw is too wide to fit into the vault of a narrow palate, the maxilla is initially widened with a nickel-titanium archwire. Depending on the age of the patient, extreme transverse expansion may require 2 rounds of expansion with RPEs.

If additional widening with a multisegment LeFort I osteotomy is needed during orthognathic surgery, the transverse width needs to be postsurgically maintained with either an acrylic plate or transpalatal arches (TPA). An acrylic palatal plate, based on the plaster model used to make the surgical splint, can be placed after the surgical splints are removed. It can maintain the transverse dimension but will limit maxillary tooth movement. Alternatively, a TPA can be placed into the lingual sheaths of the maxillary first molars to maintain maxillary molar width. This approach requires prewelding of lingual sheaths onto molar bands before the surgery. If neither the acrylic plate nor the TPA were prepared, then class III elastics

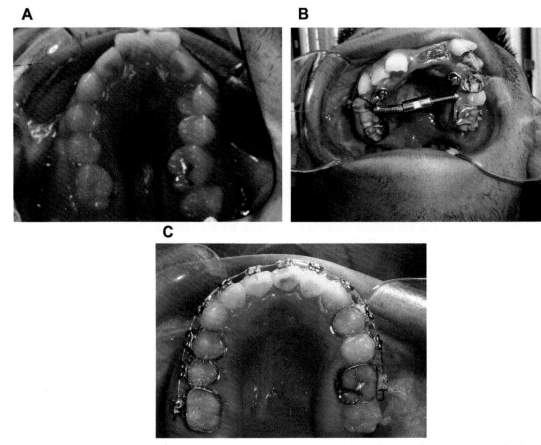

**Fig. 11.** (*A*) Distorted and narrow transverse width in a patient with a lateral facial cleft. (*B*) Extreme widening of the maxilla with a telescopic expander and an SARPE supported by intermaxillary fixation screws. (*C*) Expanded archform.

should be run from the palatal hook of the maxillary first molars to the lower buccal canine hook. When the elastics cross the occlusal table, there is an outward force placed on the maxillary molars because of a difference in transverse width of the upper molars and lower canines. This modified position of the class III elastic can help resist transverse relapse of the maxillary segments.

## ADDRESSING THE CLASS III MALOCCLUSION

In cleft lip and palate patients, the mandible is usually unaffected by the cleft and grows normally; however, the maxilla (upper jaw) often does not grow as far forward and downward as the maxilla of the noncleft child,[17] resulting in a short maxilla and a class III malocclusion (underbite). The scar contracture that occurs from the hard palate repair is thought to distort the growth of the maxilla, resulting in maxillary hypoplasia.[17–19] Fibrosis results from the stripped periosteum and affects the vertical, transverse, and AP growth of the maxilla. In addition, the fibrosis that results from

the cleft lip repair is also thought to play a role in the maxillary deficiency.[18,19] Canine substitution of the missing lateral incisor is associated with orthognathic surgery at the end of pubertal growth.[20] Approximately 22% to 59.4% of cleft lip and palate patients will need orthognathic (jaw) surgery at the end of adolescent growth to correct the maxillary deficiency.[21,22] Early treatment of class III malocclusions can reduce the need to 10%.[23]

For skeletal underbite with a difference in upper and lower jaw lengths, the standard of care is to surgically advance the maxillary bone and dentition in cleft patients with a LeFort 1 osteotomy after adolescent growth has completed, sometimes in combination with mandibular and midfacial surgeries. The advantages to surgical advancement of the upper jaw is that surgery targets bony correction, corrects the bite, and can effect a significant facial change in patients with cleft lip and palate. The cost for orthognathic surgery is expensive and is more difficult to perform in cleft patients with class III malocclusions than in noncleft patients with class III malocclusions, because of the scarring from previous surgeries, which restricts the forward and downward movement of the maxilla. Furthermore, the scarring may also increase the relapse rate associated with maxillary surgical advancement in cleft patients. Rates of relapse in these patients have been reported to occur 5% to 80% of the time.[24,25] Therefore, the patient with cleft lip and palate may go through the morbidity associated with orthognathic surgery and still relapse to the prior class III malocclusion. **Fig. 1** illustrates such a case. Because the AP difference between the maxilla and mandible exceeds 10 mm, different surgical techniques, such as distraction osteogenesis, may be needed to produce bone at the osteotomy site in cases where the amount of LeFort I bony overlap is inadequate to stably advance the maxilla large distances.

Most class III malocclusions in patients with cleft lip and palate are corrected with LeFort 1 maxillary advancement as part of the surgical plan. The analysis of a patient with cleft lip and palate shares some features like the cephalometric analysis with the noncleft patient, and the goals of treatment are similar, but the building blocks are different because there is a cleft that once divided the cleft segments and could be used for a segmental osteotomy.[26,27] The range of the maxillary advancement depends on complete mobilization of the maxilla; in practice, the maxilla should be gradually loosened so that it can be pulled into the splint position with a cotton plier. Two-jaw surgery that combines maxillary advancement with a mandibular setback and clockwise rotation of the occlusal plane can increase the range of class III correction by splitting the AP difference between the maxilla and mandible; however, the facial esthetics and cephalometric radiographs will decide whether to advance the maxilla a long distance or to split the difference between the maxilla and mandible. In these difficult cases of cleft lip and palate and class III malocclusion, the guiding principles should be whether the outcomes are achievable, stable, and esthetic.[28]

In recent years, virtual surgical planning made possible the fabrication of custom 3D-printed surgical plates that are more rigid and better adapted to the bony anatomy than surgical plates bent during surgery and are used as an aid to prevent surgical relapse. Other strategies include earlier orthopedic protraction treatment to reduce the AP discrepancy and distraction osteogenesis when the discrepancy is greater than 10 mm. **Table 1** describes the different methods that can be used to address the class III malocclusion. Because every surgical intervention has both benefit and cost/advantages and disadvantages, some of these properties are included in **Table 1**. The rigid external distractor[2] for maxillary distraction has certain advantages over the internal distractor because it can be reloaded and distracted to any length and can overcorrect a class III malocclusion. The vector of maxillary lengthening can be guided by changing the angle and point of attachment for the connecting wires. However, the patient must be willing to wear a visible RED halo for 3 months. Showing the patient before and after photographs from previous cases corrected by the RED devices can help with patient acceptance. Internal distractors have the advantage of being partially hidden, but the activating arms that exit the oral cavity can impinge on the inner lip or cheek during lengthening, thereby producing a painful ulceration in the mucosa. One modification has been to reverse the orientation of the distractor arm so that the distractor arms exit behind the ear. Bilateral internal distractors also require the placement of either an RPE[29] or a transpalatal acrylic plate to prevent the cleft segments from being torn apart by separate distractors that are placed along the side of the maxilla in a convergent vector due to the shape of the maxilla. Finally, one of the drawbacks to both maxillary protraction and distraction techniques is the inability to correct maxillary yaw because it is difficult to rotate the maxilla during the distraction process. A final LeFort 1 surgery may be needed at the time of distractor removal to correct the midline and residual class III malocclusion.

If the patient is seen during childhood or early adolescence, then orthopedic approaches like maxillary protraction can be used to lessen the severity of a class III malocclusion and reduce the need for orthognathic surgery.[30] If done too early, then the class III malocclusion can return during adolescence because of the growth of the mandible. If done too late, the sutures may fuse, making the treatment difficult to carry out or become less stable. At Children's Hospital Los Angeles, a multicenter study clinical trial is being conducted to compare surgical and protraction techniques to correct the class III malocclusion in patients with cleft lip and palate. The authors' sutural loosening protocol is as follows: at age 11 to 14, the maxilla is loosened by alternating a week of RPE expansion with a week of constriction for 8 weeks before applying class III elastics during the daytime and reverse-pull facemask protraction elastics during the evening. The correction of the underbite may occur through a combination of skeletal, dentoalveolar, and occlusal changes. Similarly, in Bauru, Brazil, the

**Table 1**
**Surgical orthodontic class III solutions**

| Procedure | Benefit | Disadvantages |
|---|---|---|
| >10 mm of AP correction | | |
| RED distraction-rigid external device | Overcorrection, midfacial correction | Psychosocial effect of visible halo |
| Bilateral maxillary internal distraction-intraoral device | Finish correction with LeFort I osteotomy, splints, and plates during distractor removal, less visible | Undercorrection, pressure ulcerations to maxillary cheek and lip |
| LeFort I distraction with Bollard plates/class III elastics and facemask | Quick recovery, comfortable, invisible, TADs can also be used | Depends on patient cooperation |
| Staged LeFort I performed twice with bilateral sagittal split osteotomy (BSSO) | No distraction problems; precise occlusion | Two orthognathic surgeries |
| LeFort III/LeFort I | Midfacial correction and occlusal correction | Increased risks of intracranial surgery |
| LeFort III/distract LeFort II by cutting zygoma after Le Fort III | Effective method for LeFort II distraction when needed | Large surgery with risks, can increase airway and increase vertical by clockwise rotation |
| Anterior segmental distraction | Quick recovery, treats relapse and dental crowding | Custom distractor, segmental cuts, edentulous distraction site |
| LeFort I/BSSO/malar implants | Camouflage | Compromise esthetics if problem is short maxilla |
| 7–10 mm | | |
| LeFort I, anterior nasal spine wedge dissection as needed | Targets where the skeletal deficiency is | Limited by bony overlap in AP direction, less stable than BSSO setback due to less bony contact |
| Up to 6 mm, protraction techniques during early adolescence | | |
| Bollard plates with class III elastics | Temporomandibular joint remodels, few dentoalveolar effects, can avoid orthognathic surgery | 5 y of elastic wear, difficult to correct maxillary midlines, Bollard plates loosen, depends on cooperation |
| Alternate expansion/ constriction, sutural loosening with facemask and class III elastics/Essix retainers and canine brackets or with protraction spring | Can avoid orthognathic surgery, improves maxillary incisor inclination | More dentoalveolar effects, counterclockwise rotation of occlusal plane, may relapse, difficult to correct maxillary midline, depends on cooperation |
| Less than 3 mm anterior crossbite | | |
| Lower bicuspid extraction | Avoids second surgery, mandibular correction, uprights lower incisors | Dental compensation, compromise esthetics if maxilla relapses |
| MEAW with class III and anterior vertical elastics | Distalization mechanics that uprights entire dentition, mandibular correction | Lower third molars must be extracted, depends on patient cooperation, can worsen without compliance |
| TAD supported distalization of lower dentition | May avoid reoperation, avoids premolar extraction, less cooperation needed | Difficult to accomplish due to posterior interferences, third molars must be extracted, TADs can loosen |

(continued on next page)

**Table 1**
**(*continued*)**

| Procedure | Benefit | Disadvantages |
|---|---|---|
| Anterior segmental distraction | Corrects maxillary relapse, treats crowding and improves incisor display | Small surgery, short recovery period, potential damage to dental roots if not prepared |
| TPA/class III elastics from palatal hooks | Maintains postsurgical correction, corrects upper molar torque | Requires placement of lingual sheaths |

Bollard plate is used for maxillary protraction[27] by attaching skeletal plates to the maxilla above the first molar and to the mandible below the canine and lateral incisors. The plates transmit the elastic forces directly to the basal bone, and therefore, have less dentoalveolar changes. Twelve years ago, Bollard plates were used in combination with a LeFort I surgery at Children's Hospital Los Angeles in order to distract the maxilla by elastic tension. The correction by elastic maxillary distraction is more rapid than maxillary protraction but depends on patient cooperation. If a surgery is needed to place and remove the Bollard plates, then a surgery that is similar to an SARPE or incomplete LeFort I osteotomy could be done at the same time to distract the maxilla. The down fracture of the pterygoid plates is incomplete and leaves a small amount of bone to stabilize the LeFort I segment to form a callus during the latency period. The down fracture is completed by the elastic tension on the osteotomized maxilla. If the maxilla is completely separated during surgery, then the maxilla should be held against the host bone during the latency period by placing intermaxillary fixation screws above and below the osteotomy and keeping the segments together with surgical wire or sutures that are removed 3 days later. Alternatively, the patient can wear a vertical chin-cup for 3 days to hold the maxillary segments against the host bone above it during the latency period.

## RELAPSE AND RETENTION

TADs and Bollard plates can play an important role for guiding distraction procedures, assist in postsurgical segmental adjustments, and provide anchorage for orthodontic tooth movement. It can also be used to prevent relapse of the skeletal correction after the surgery has been completed. **Fig. 12** shows a sequence of cephalometric radiographs that illustrate how residents bought the wrong hardware for RED distraction and created an open bite.[31] To correct the open bite, TADs were placed in the mandible and maxilla, and then the maxilla was surgically loosened. Wire loops connected the TADs to the archwire so that interarch elastics for closing the open bite would not extrude teeth; rather, the elastic forces were transmitted to the bone by the wires connecting the TAD to the archwire. After the open bite was largely corrected, a surgical splint was constructed for a final LeFort 1 osteotomy and placed during distractor removal in order to obtain final correction of the class III malocclusion.

Regardless of the method used to correct the class III malocclusion, treatment relapse is a possibility in the patient with cleft lip and palate; therefore, the struggle for stability during the postsurgical and retention period can be aided by class III elastics. If surgical relapse occurs, the class III malocclusion can be addressed by moving the mandibular dentition distally or by distracting the anterior maxilla. If the lower incisors are proclined, then an orthodontic option is to extract the lower first bicuspids and retract the lower anterior teeth by uprighting the incisors. If the surgery relapses to an edge-to-edge class III malocclusion, then nonextraction multiloop edgewise archwire (MEAW) mechanics[32] can be used to upright the lower incisors and correct a class III malocclusion provided the lower third molars were extracted before surgery and the lower incisors can tolerate uprighting. The entire mandibular dentition is distalized along a multilooped archwire that is bent in a reverse curve (**Fig. 13**). The class III and vertical elastics used with MEAW can anchor the lower incisors so that the archwire acts like a giant spring to distalize and intrude the second molars. If the patient is noncompliant, then the class III malocclusion will worsen. If the patient does not wear the elastics needed for MEAW mechanics, then a TAD placed mesial to the mandibular molar or near the first premolar can be used to support a pull coil spring from the TAD.

For retention, an Essix retainer with class III hooks is used with class III elastics during the first year after appliances are removed.

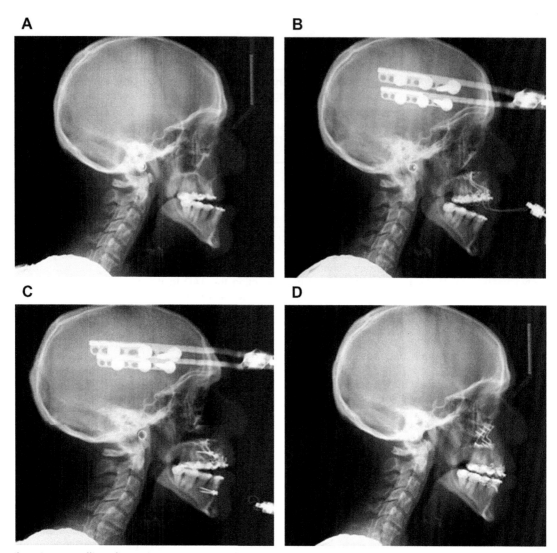

**Fig. 12.** Controlling distraction outcomes with TADs. (*A*) Presurgical cephalometric radiograph. (*B*) Incorrect distraction vector due to L-plate attachment to RED instead of wire. (*C*) Screws placed to close open bite without extruding teeth. Wire loop for TAD to archwire transmitted interarch elastic force to the TAD. (*D*) At the time of distractor removal, final correction was attained with a LeFort 1 osteotomy with surgical plates and splint. (*From Yen SLK, Late maxillary protraction techniques for cleft lip and palate. Semin Orthod. 2017;23:307; with permission.*)

## DISCUSSION

Patients with cleft lip and palate are often treated using the same types of cephalometric analyses and the surgical approaches as the noncleft patient. There are many treatment goals that are shared between these 2 groups of patients, such as good speech and hearing, a stable and functional occlusion, good periodontal health of the dentition, correction of dental midlines, minimal scarring and facial asymmetries, and good display of the maxillary incisors and canines. However, the cleft anatomy poses additional problems to

correct, especially in patients with large cleft lip and palate defects, and not all the goals are perfectly achievable. Each procedure has both a benefit and a disadvantage so the team has to choose their priorities as to which goals to work on based on the chief complaints as well as knowledge of growth and development. For the treatment of complex and difficult cases, a one-protocol-to-fit-all-patients approach may not solve all of the problems with which the patient presents. Each cleft is different as are the set of problems associated with the cleft. The more extensive a facial cleft is, the harder it is to imagine

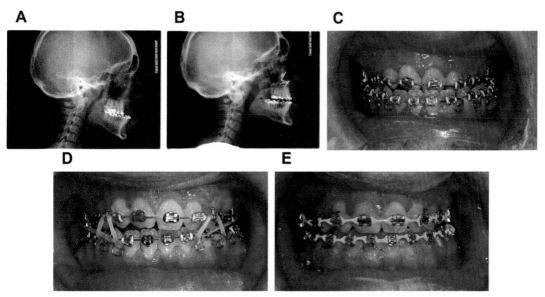

**Fig. 13.** Correction of surgical relapse. (*A*) Presurgical cephalometric radiograph. (*B*) Postsurgical radiograph. (*C*) Postsurgical relapse into class III malocclusion after maxillary distraction and a LeFort I maxillary surgery. (*D*) MEAW wires were placed to correct class III malocclusion with class III and vertical elastics. (*E*) Correction obtained by a cooperative patient who wore continuous elastics for 2 months.

what the repaired face and jaws should look like. Cephalometric proportionate template analyses like Moorrees,[33] Jacobson,[34] Burlington,[35] and Bolton[36] analyses can help to superimpose the overall shape of an average face over the patient's facial skeleton and help make sense of unusual angular and linear measurements. A presurgical CT scan should be taken to trace the extent and size of the cleft defect and provide clues on how the different bones collapsed into the void of the cleft. Reversing the direction of vertical, horizontal, and AP collapse can help the clinician picture what a face without a cleft might have looked like and help establish treatment goals.[37] The surgeries for the complex cases of cleft lip and palate often resemble reconstructive strategies used to treat facial fractures. The decision to follow one strategy over another should be based on achievability, stability, and facial esthetics.

It is hoped, by late adolescence, that the patient with cleft lip and palate will not need orthognathic surgery or have few difficult problems to address. The goal of earlier surgeries is to help minimize the remaining problems in the late adolescent patient. Currently, several intercenter comparison studies[38,39] are being conducted to find the best overall cleft-related protocols. In Europe, certain countries limit cleft lip and palate surgeries to a small number of surgeons and centers with high-volume surgeons to ensure a high standard and quality of care.[40] This strategy is indeed a way to raise the level of national care for patients with cleft lip and palate

but requires national policy making and can work within countries with socialized medicine where the costs of care are covered by society. There is a clear benefit, but there is also a cost. In the United States, it is difficult to centralize care, to receive compensation to cover the cost for craniofacial care, to standardize care using national protocols, and to limit the care to national centers with only a few chosen surgeons while addressing the unmet need of craniofacial care for the entire US population. In a national health care system, the number of fellowship and teaching programs might be limited in order to prevent inexperienced surgeons and orthodontists from working on patients with cleft lip and palate. The debate on how to best provide care should start with discussions on best practices at a national level and on training requirements for fellowship training programs. Despite the best efforts to raise the overall care of patients within a national health care system or within a hospital or university, in an urban environment, there will remain patients who need complex care. These patients are the ones with unusually large cleft defects or who were treated for their primary surgeries in less-developed countries. Moreover, these patients might not be able to be successfully treated using standardized protocols, so the criteria for trying out an alternative protocol needs to be examined. When a standardized or traditional, one-size-fit-all protocol fails, then it becomes necessary to reanalyze the case and to think of changes that can address the unresolved clinical problem with which the patient presents. This article was written to share some different strategies that were used to address these complex cases and is presented to help craniofacial teams with their decision-making process as they undertake the orthodontics and surgery needed to treat complex cleft lip and palate cases during late adolescence.

## ACKNOWLEDGMENTS

The distraction strategies were developed from research studies support by the American Association of Oral and Maxillofacial Surgeons, the American Association of Orthodontists Foundation and the Chalmer J. Lyons Academy. The late maxillary protraction and orthognathic surgery outcomes were studied under a research grant from the NIDCR:UO1DE022937-06.

## DISCLOSURE

The authors have nothing to disclose.

## REFERENCES

1. ACPA parameters for evaluation and treatment of patients with cleft lip/palate or other craniofacial differences. Cleft Palate Craniofac J 2018;55(1): 137–56.
2. Sant'Anna EF, Cury-Saramago Ade A, Lau GW, et al. Treatment of midfacial hypoplasia in syndromic and cleft lip and palate patients by means of a rigid external distractor (RED). Dental Press J Orthod 2013;18(4):134–43.
3. Lypka M, Afshar A, Pham D, et al. Implant-supported distraction osteogenesis: a technique to advance the deficient maxilla. J Craniofac Surg 2009;20(2):525–7.
4. Tanikawa C, Lee D, Oonishi YY, et al. The elimination of dental crowding and development of a proper dental arch by maxillary anterior segmental distraction osteogenesis for a patient with UCLP. Cleft Palate Craniofac J 2019;56(7): 978–85.
5. Palermo A. Master's thesis, detrimental effect of dental encroachment on secondary alveolar bone graft outcomes in the treatment of patients with cleft lip and palate. Los Angeles (CA): University of Southern California; 2019.
6. Dissaux C, Bodin F, Grollemund B, et al. Evaluation of success of alveolar cleft bone graft performed at 5 years versus 10 years of age. J Craniomaxillofac Surg 2016;44(1):21–6.
7. Fahradyan A, Tsuha M, Wolfswinkel EM, et al. Optimal timing of secondary alveolar bone grafting: a literature review. J Oral Maxillofac Surg 2019; 77(4):843–9.
8. Vachiramon A, Urata M, Kyung HM, et al. Clinical applications of orthodontic microimplant anchorage in craniofacial patients. Am J Orthod Dentofacial Orthop 2009;136(6):770.e1-11.
9. Yen SL, Gross J, Wang P, et al. Closure of a large alveolar cleft by bony transport of a posterior segment using orthodontic archwires attached to bone: report of a case. J Oral Maxillofac Surg 2001;59(6):688–91.
10. Yen SL, Yamashita DD, Kim TH, et al. Closure of an unusually large palatal fistula in a cleft patient by bony transport and corticotomy-assisted expansion. J Oral Maxillofac Surg 2003;61(11):1346–50.
11. Yen SL, Yamashita DD, Gross J, et al. Combining orthodontic tooth movement with distraction osteogenesis to close cleft spaces and improve maxillary arch form in cleft lip and palate patients. Am J Orthod Dentofacial Orthop 2005;127(2): 224–32.
12. Suzuki A, Nakano M, Yoshizaki K, et al. A longitudinal study of the presence of dental anomalies in the primary and permanent dentitions of cleft lip and/or palate patients. Cleft Palate Craniofac J 2017;54(3): 309–20.
13. Torres A, AlYazeedy I, Yen S. A programmable expander for patients with cleft lip and palate. Cleft Palate Craniofac J 2019;56(6):837–44.
14. Zachrisson BU. On current trends in adult treatment, part 2. Interview by Robert G. Keim. J Clin Orthod 2005;39(5):285–96.
15. Lee MK, Lane C, Azeredo F, et al. Clinical effectiveness of late maxillary protraction in cleft lip and palate: a methods paper. Orthod Craniofac Res 2017; 20(Suppl 1):129–33.
16. Vargervik K. Growth characteristics of the premaxilla and orthodontic treatment principles in bilateral cleft lip and palate. Cleft Palate J 1983;20(4):289–302.
17. Liao YF, Mars M. Long-term effects of palate repair on craniofacial morphology in patients with unilateral cleft lip and palate. Cleft Palate Craniofac J 2005; 42(6):594–600.
18. Mars M, Houston WJ. A preliminary study of facial growth and morphology in unoperated male unilateral cleft lip and palate subjects over 13 years of age. Cleft Palate J 1990;27(1):7–10.
19. Ross RB. Treatment variables affecting facial growth in complete unilateral cleft lip and palate. Cleft Palate J 1987;24(1):5–77.
20. Lee JC, Slack GC, Walker R, et al. Maxillary hypoplasia in the cleft patient: contribution of orthodontic dental space closure to orthognathic surgery. Plast Reconstr Surg 2014;133(2): 355–61.
21. Good PM, Mulliken JB, Padwa BL. Frequency of Le-Fort I osteotomy after repaired cleft lip and palate or cleft palate. Cleft Palate Craniofac J 2007;44(4): 396–401.

22. Daskalogiannakis J, Mehta M. The need for orthognathic surgery in patients with repaired complete unilateral and complete bilateral cleft lip and palate. Cleft Palate Craniofac J 2009;46(5): 498–502.

23. Oberoi S, Hoffman WY, Chigurupati R, et al. Frequency of surgical correction for maxillary hypoplasia in cleft lip and palate. J Craniofac Surg 2012; 23(6):166.

24. Baek SH, Lee JK, Lee JH, et al. Comparison of treatment outcome and stability between distraction osteogenesis and LeFort I osteotomy in cleft patients with maxillary hypoplasia. J Craniofac Surg 2007; 18(5):1209–15.

25. Rachmiel A. Treatment of maxillary cleft palate: distraction osteogenesis versus orthognathic surgery–part one: maxillary distraction. J Oral Maxillofac Surg 2007;65(4):753–7.

26. Posnick JC, Tompson B. Cleft-orthognathic surgery: complications and long-term results. Plast Reconstr Surg 1995;96(2):255–66.

27. Posnick JC. The treatment of secondary and residual dentofacial deformities in the cleft patient. Surgical and orthodontic therapy. Clin Plast Surg 1997; 24(3):583–97.

28. Rachmiel A, Even-Almos M, Aizenbud D. Treatment of maxillary cleft palate: distraction osteogenesis vs. orthognathic surgery. Ann Maxillofac Surg 2012; 2(2):127–30.

29. Lypka M, Yen S, Urata M, et al. Solving convergent vector problems with internal maxillary distractors through the use of a fixed rapid palatal expander. J Oral Maxillofac Surg 2012;70(7):e428–30.

30. Tindlund RS. Orthopaedic protraction of the midface in the deciduous dentition. Results covering 3 years out of treatment. J Craniomaxillofac Surg 1989; 17(Suppl 1):17–9.

31. Yen SLK. Late maxillary protraction techniques for cleft lip and palate. Semin Orthod 2017;23:305–13.

32. Baek SH, Shin SJ, Ahn SJ, et al. Initial effect of multiloop edgewise archwire on the mandibular dentition in class III malocclusion subjects. A three-dimensional finite element study. Eur J Orthod 2008;30(1):10–5.

33. Ghafari J. Modified use of the Moorrees mesh diagram analysis. Am J Orthod Dentofacial Orthop 1987;91(6):475–82.

34. Jacobson A. Orthognathic diagnosis using the proportionate template. J Oral Surg 1980;38(11): 820–33.

35. Popovich F, Thompson GW. Craniofacial templates for orthodontic case analysis. Am J Orthod 1977; 71(4):406–20.

36. Hans MG, Broadbent BH, Nelson S. Broadbent-Bolton growth study–past, present, and future. Am J Orthod Dentofacial Orthop 1994;106: 598–603.

37. David DJ, Moore MH, Cooter RD. Tessier clefts revisited with a third dimension. Cleft Palate J 1989;26(3): 163–84.

38. Long RE, Shaw WC, Semb G. Eurocleft and the Americleft studies. An experiment in intercenter and international collaboration. Cleft lip and palate. Diagnosis and management. 3rd edition. Berlin: Springer Nature; 2013.

39. Shaw WC, Semb G, Nelson P, et al. The Eurocleft project 1996–2000: overview. J Craniomaxillofac Surg 2001;29(3):131–40.

40. Fitzsimmons KJ, Mukarram S, Copley LP, et al. Centralisation of services for children with cleft lip or palate in England: a study of hospital episode statistics. BMC Health Serv Res 2012;12:148.

# LeFort Distraction in the Cleft Patient

Stephanie J. Drew, DMD[a],*, Hitesh Kapadia, DDS, PhD[b]

**KEYWORDS**

- Le Fort • Distraction • Cleft

**KEY POINTS**

- Indications for DO in the cleft patient.
- Orthodontic considerations for LeFort DO.
- Protocol for planning this surgery virtually.
- The indications and uses for Internal versus external distraction devices.

## HISTORY OF MAXILLARY DISTRACTION IN THE CLEFT PATIENT VIA LeFort I OSTEOTOMY

Distraction osteogenesis (DO) was originally described as a way to lengthen the limbs by Codavilla in 1905.[1] The technique was later refined by Ilizarov as a technique to lengthen long bones, presenting the tenets to use an appropriate rate and rhythm of advancement of the devices for distraction.[2,3] A comprehensive review of the biology of bone formation and fracture healing, as well as distraction osteogenesis, can be found in the 2017 paper by Runyan and Gabrick.[4] DO was first applied to the mandible of a human craniofacial skeleton. In 1992 McCarthy and colleagues[5] published their paper on DO in the craniofacial skeleton by applying the technique to the mandible in a patient with hemifacial microsomia, after which work began in the craniofacial population to see if DO could be applied in the midface and maxilla.

Maxillary DO was first described by using dog and sheep experiments, respectively, by Block and Brister[6] on dog anterior maxillary DO (AMD) in 1994 and by Rachmiel and colleagues[7] on sheep using internal distractors and total LeFort DO (TMD) in 1993. In 1995, Cohen and colleagues[8] reported on the use of DO to advance the maxilla using Internal devices in humans. These techniques were later modified by Polley and Figueroa[9] in 1997 using external devices to achieve better 3D control of the movement, especially in craniofacial syndromes. Since then, various modifications of these devices have been made, as well as indications, protocols, and timing of the technique.[10] Because the technique not only allows for bone growth but also the stretching of tissues, its use has been adopted by many cleft surgeons for use in cleft patients with severe maxillary hypoplasia.

## TYPES OF MAXILLARY DISTRACTION DEVICES
### External Devices

The external devices were the first distractors used for 3D control and are still used today to move the maxilla and midface primarily in very complex craniofacial patients. There is a cranial halo anchor that is secured to the skull with pins and the midline vertical member bar, which has mobile horizontal bars that can move along (up and down) the length of these devices to provide anchorage for the wires that will be attached to the distractor plates or to the orthodontic modified hyrax anchors (**Fig. 1**). The screws attached to these horizontal bars are tightened at a specific rate and rhythm and the wires are then shortened thus bringing the maxilla forward. The typical rate

[a] Department of Surgery, Division of Oral and Maxillofacial Surgery, Emory University School of Medicine, 1365 Clifton Road Northeast, Building B, Suite 2300, Atlanta, GA 30322, USA; [b] Craniofacial Orthodontics, Seattle Children's Hospital, Craniofacial Center, M/S OB.9.520, 4800 Sand Point Way Northeast, Seattle, WA 98105, USA
* Corresponding author.
E-mail address: Stephanie.drew@emory.edu

Oral Maxillofacial Surg Clin N Am 32 (2020) 269–281
https://doi.org/10.1016/j.coms.2020.01.010

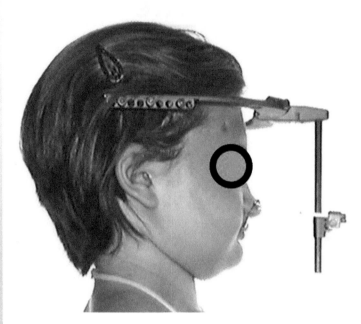

**Fig. 1.** Rigid external distraction (RED) external distractor in position.

is 1 mm per day of forward movement. The best advantage for these appliances is that the vectors can be altered while moving the bones forward. When moving the facial skeleton of a severe craniofacial patient, such as a child with Cruzon syndrome, this is of utmost importance because the vectors are complex.

The disadvantage of these devices is that if only a simple movement in any direction needs to be made, they are cumbersome and difficult to wear in public and go to school and socialize. There is also the risk of intracranial penetration/migration of the halo pins, which can become a neurosurgical emergency and must be dealt with promptly.[11–14]

### Internal Devices

The need for less cumbersome devices to be developed has led to miniaturization of the distraction screws such that they could be placed intraorally and hidden. These devices are limited by the size of the lengthening screws to advance the maxilla and the strength of the devices as they are lengthened. The advent of the telescoping lengthening screws has compensated for this problem. The internal devices are also limited because they are unidirectional. Thus, planning vectors is difficult because they must be placed bilaterally. The advent of virtual planning and consideration to have customization of the devices has helped a great deal with gaining predictable movement of the maxilla along the correct vector.

Submerged multidirectional devices have been attempted and are bulky, very cumbersome, and difficult to place and manipulate. These devices also require adequate bone stock for anchorage superiorly and at times inferiorly (**Fig. 2**). Often the lower arm of the distractor is anchored to modifications of the orthodontic appliances attached to the dentition (**Fig. 3**).

Of note, in the pediatric patient with mixed dentition, the area to place the lower moving plate is limited by the developing dentition. The use of tooth-borne anchorage devices should also be considered in these cases to prevent developing teeth from being damaged.

A comparison of the use of external devices versus internal devices can be found in 2008

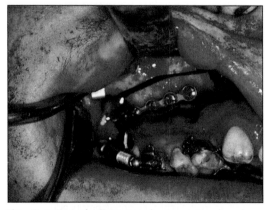

**Fig. 2.** Intraoral distractor lower arm placed on adequate bone stock below osteotomy.

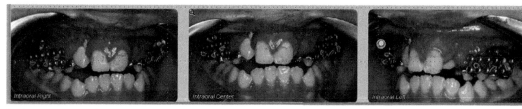

**Fig. 3.** Devices in place and wired to lower orthodontic appliances.

clinical controversies papers by Figueroa and Polley (part I) and Drew (part II).[15,16]

## TYPES OF ANCHORAGE

For the internal distractors, the superior portion of the distractor is placed and stabilized with screws into the zygoma. The lower member is then attached to either the maxillary bone above the roots but below the LeFort cut (see **Fig. 2**) or to an appliance that is secured to the lower teeth appliance modification (see **Fig. 3**). The external devices again are anchored to the skull with bone screws to hold it in place and the maxilla is connected with bone plates either directly to the bone or to an appliance attached to the teeth.

## BONE BORNE DISTRACTOR DEVICES

The cleft maxilla that needs distraction is hypoplastic in 3 dimensions. The bone stock available may be deficient to the point that there is no room to place the lower bone plate arm and screws of the distractor without placing them into tooth roots. This is also true in the young patient requiring distraction with developing dentition. In these cases, bonded hyrax appliances are useful to attach the lower member to welded loops on the hyrax device (**Fig. 4**).

## COMBINATION BONE TO TOOTH BORNE

These devices can be connected to the teeth with either bands connected with a modified hyrax device or with a modified bonded occlusal hyrax that has the ability to allow for the lower member of the distraction arm to be attached with wires. This type of combined anchorage may also be used in AMD; however, it is recommended to use complete bone-borne devices for pushing the anterior maxillary segment.[17–19]

## TRANSPALATAL SUPPORT IN THE CLEFT PALATE PATIENT

Despite grafting of the alveolar cleft defect the hard palate is only soft tissue. The alveolus may not be strong enough to withstand the pressures of downfracture during the LeFort I without some type of transpalatal support (**Fig. 5**). If not, the maxilla may fracture through the alveolar cleft and the distraction attempt will need to be aborted unless some type of transpalatal support can be placed.

With a tooth-borne distractor, often customizing a hyrax device will suffice for this purpose. The molar and premolar bands can be joined on the buccal surface by soldering on a wire with loops to allow for connection to the lower member of the distraction device

With bone-borne distractors, using the hyrax can also be done, especially if width may need to be obtained after advancement and consolidation.

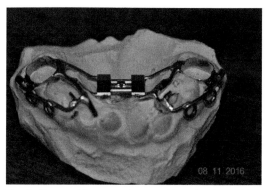

**Fig. 4.** Hyrax with custom loops soldered to lateral bar of hyrax to attach distractor lower plate arm to with wires.

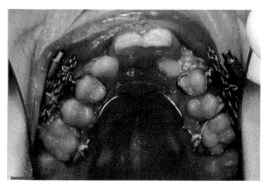

**Fig. 5.** Trans palatal support with orthodontic transpalatal wire.

## INDICATIONS FOR LeFort I DISTRACTION OSTEOGENESIS IN THE CLEFT PATIENT

LeFort distraction is used to move the severe maxillary hypoplastic maxilla in an anterior vector to correct severe maxillary anteroposterior deficiency. It can also be used to move slightly downward in trajectory, but this is not the main purpose of the technique. The technique can be considered to be used when standard osteotomy techniques would not be stable and at increased risk for relapse. In the cleft patient population, when the maxilla requires more than 10 mm of movement, as result of scar tissues and small bone stock, there is an increased risk for relapse. In 2004, Adolphs and colleagues[20] reviewed their DO work over a 10-year period for the entire craniofacial skeleton. Of note, is that they reserved using DO only for their most complicated and large maxillary movements. This was a very small percentage (1%) in their treatment of hypoplasia of the maxilla in their cleft population. Also they only used internal distractors for their LeFort movement.

## CONTRAINDICATIONS

Noncompliance of the patient and/or family plays a vital role in the success or failure of distraction surgery. Once the device is secured into position it must be activated daily by the parent, patient, or the surgical team. If the patient cannot tolerate this or refuses to cooperate, the distraction will fail and the maxilla will consolidate. Also, if the patient is noncompliant in terms of activity, say insists on going on a jungle gym and falling off, the distractors can break and perhaps be pulled out of the bone and thus causing a failure of the distraction. Even worse, with halo distractors, falling can push a pin through the cranium and into the brain resulting in a neurosurgical emergency.

The inability to carefully monitor the progress of the bone movement and consolidation may lead to failure. When a patient presents for care who may live in a very remote area, it is difficult to monitor the progress of the distractor turning and maxillary movement. Telemedicine may be adequate in some situations. However, an adequate follow-up plan must be discussed and committed to well in advance of the surgery; perhaps also educating a team closer to home to help out with this part of the process may be available to the primary team.

Poor stock of bone or teeth to create anchorage for the devices can lead to failure of distraction. The distractors depend on anchoring the proximal and distal bone plates such that when the distraction rod is turned it pushes the plates apart moving the mobile piece of bone with it along the vector of placement. If the bone is of poor quality or there are no teeth for anchorage, it is difficult to use distractors.

## TIMING

Timing of distraction at the LeFort level must also be included in a discussion about indications for surgery. There are reports about the use of this technique in children under 10 years old, adolescent middle school children, and the patient who is skeletally mature. When considering the reasons why one would want to correct a significant skeletal malformation in the younger group, some of the issues to note are the psychosocial impact of this deformity, the ability of the patient to speak and close their lips, the compromised ability to masticate, and perhaps a component of breathing may be affected, such as in the patient with sleep apnea that developed after soft palate repair or pharyngeal flap surgery.

The use of LeFort DO in the growing patient is not without consequence. Liu and Zhou[21] and Doucet and colleagues[22] suggest that advancement of the maxilla must be planned such that it is over distracted by at least 15% to 25%, as there is minimal growth after the DO surgery is completed. However, when one considers using this technique as a staging surgery for future orthognathic surgery, the planning can take that into account. Think of using a procedure like SARPE (surgically assisted rapid palatal expansion) to gain anteroposterior dimension instead of width (surgically assisted rapid maxillary advancement via DO [SARMADO]). Also of note is that orthognathic surgery may still be necessary in some patients after early DO.[23]

Planning DO surgery for adult patients should aim to essentially reverse engineer the maxilla from final occlusion endpoint. Once this is determined, careful orthodontic alignment of the lower dentition, paying attention to the lower incisor angulation, will give us the goal to achieve. Alignment of the upper dentition, especially the angle of the incisors, will also give us our surgical endpoint. Once this planning is completed then the decision to use DO as a staging surgery, such as SARPE (SARMADO) or to achieve a final occlusion, can be determined.

## PROTOCOL TO PLAN LeFort DISTRACTION OSTEOGENESIS

All maxillary distraction cases must be reverse engineered. Whether using internal or external devices, we need to have a goal. Determining the final position of the maxilla and final occlusion is done with a combination of physical examination, dental models, photographs, 3D computed tomographic (CT) imaging, stereolithic models when needed, and virtual planning including cephalometric analysis. Once the final position is determined, the distractor vectors can then be chosen, as well as the choice of surgery, such as total maxillary DO, AMD, or orthognathic surgery alone. If DO is chosen and once the vector of movement is chosen the distractors can then be oriented to create this path of movement.

In 2018, Richardson and colleagues[24] developed a logical and clear protocol for decision making regarding maxillary advancement in the cleft maxilla. The process was divided along 3 time lines. The 5- to 11-year-old age group was distracted with TMD when it was severe; otherwise face mask therapy was used. The 11- to 16-year-old age group was divided into mild, moderate, and severe. The mild and moderate group had AMD only preserving the molar relationship and decreasing the risk of velopharyngeal incompetence (VPI). The severe group needed up to 2 AMDs owing to limitations of the advancement screws or TMD.

In the groups of 16 year and older, once growth was almost complete the mild group had standard orthognathic surgery, the moderate group with VPI had AMD, and the moderate group without VPI had orthognathic surgery. The severe group had AMD twice if positive for VPI, as before, or TMD.

In the cases listed above, careful collaboration with the orthodontic team is needed to help establish the goal occlusion and to help the patient be orthodontically optimized as far as incisor angulation as well as creating cross-arch stability.

With internal distractors, special consideration must be given to the orientation of the long axis of the arms to the vector from a 3D and also a bilateral standpoint (**Fig. 6**). One must especially take into account the orientation of the distractors in the sagittal plane. The distractors should be as parallel to one another as possible so that the device will not be blocked out and bind along the length of the screw preventing further advancement of the maxilla (**Fig. 7**). If they are not oriented properly they can also impinge on the facial labial soft tissues and may even create pressure necrosis (**Fig. 8**). The more parallel the distractor arms become in the sagittal plane, the more they may impinge on the soft tissues of the lip and midface.

The possibility of customizing the distractor to the correct vector is now possible owing to virtual planning and 3D printing. One must realize that the maxilla will not be able to move in a straight line to achieve the endpoint. Internal distractors typically move in only one direction or plane. Reflecting back on the tenets of proper distraction, an osteotomy is created, the device is placed and checked to make sure it will move along the planned path, a latency of 7 days occurs to allow for the beginning of fracture healing, then the device is active at 1 mm per day, usually in divided 0.5-mm movements; once docked it is in the consolidation phase until bone healing occurs (**Figs. 9** and **10**).

If we are to reverse engineer the movement along the planned vector, then home base (or the start point) is truly going to have to be different from the uncut maxillary position to allow this to work properly and not create a malocclusion. However, the bone position has to allow for development of a distraction chamber between the cut edges of the bones during the latency period. This positioning will sometimes require placement of either an intermediate type of splint to orient the maxilla to this new starting point or predictive holes when using a custom (patient specific) device.

Ultimately, a stereolithic model is most helpful to prebend the distractors to the correct vector if custom plates and drill guides are not used. Occlusal-based orientation guides can be used to orient the distraction screw on the model, then the arms can be bent to the bone and if needed the lateral hyrax soldered loops or lower part of the osteotomy (depending if the case will be bone or tooth borne).

The setup for the use of external DO devices is a bit less cumbersome; however, reverse engineering goals should also be used to plan out the final occlusion to be achieved. The device will be connected to the cranium and either the bone directly and/or an appliance that is cemented to the dentition (**Fig. 11**). The connector to the appliance must be made to keep the pressure off the lips to prevent necrosis (**Fig. 12**).

## ORTHODONTIC TREATMENT PROTOCOL

The orthodontic team has the responsibility to help plan and guide the distraction process with the surgeon. Predistraction orthodontics, orthodontic manipulation during DO and the consolidation phase, post-DO orthodontic management, and retention are all phases to consider when planning.[25,26]

Orthodontic alignment of the dentition is done to prepare to reverse engineer the plan from the goal of surgery in the adult patient. The preparation is essentially the same as preparing to decompensate for any class III skeletal malocclusion. Taking out compensations and rotations and leveling the

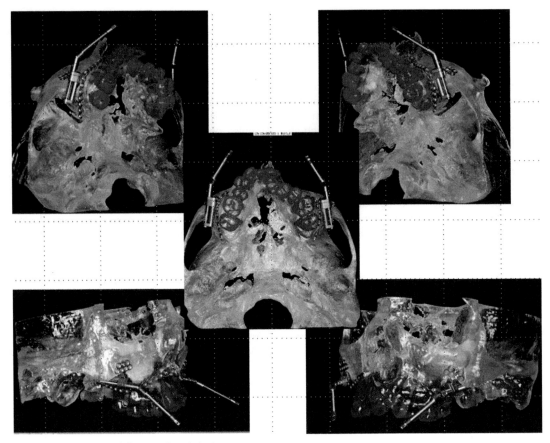

**Fig. 6.** Stereolithic models to prebend devices to correct vector.

occlusal planes when indicated with the aim of maximizing the skeletal correction. The orthodontic appliances are very helpful to use with interarch guiding elastics if needed as the bone is moving forward; also, passive rectangular arch wires with surgical hooks to engage interarch elastics. Another helpful appliance is a smooth guide plane occlusal splint on the mandible so that the maxilla will not be "caught" within the maxillary arch as it moves forward. In addition, root divergence is

**Fig. 7.** Virtual surgical planning (VSP) showing correct orientation of distractor arms bilaterally.

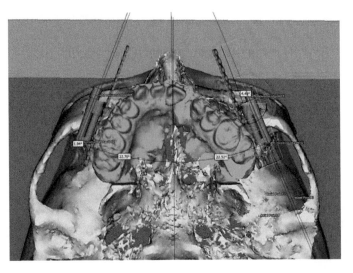

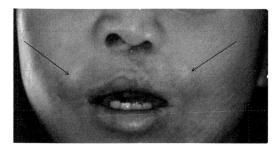

**Fig. 8.** Intraoral distractor arms creating pressure.

needed for interdental osteotomies if AMD is to be used.

Although this setup is helpful, it is not mandatory, because predicting the remaining skeletal growth in the growing patient is difficult. Most likely these children will require a secondary surgery to correct the skeletal misalignment after growth is completed.

What is mandatory, however, is the use of transpalatal support during DO in the cleft maxilla. Although the alveolar bone graft may be consolidated across the complete cleft lip and palate, the bone stock itself may not tolerate the pressures generated by the distractors and can lead to a pathologic fracture through the alveolar bone. This instability will lead to loosening of the screws in the maxilla and failure of the devices. For this reason transpalatal support is so essential when distracting a cleft maxilla. The authors recommend the use of a hyrax as a transpalatal support bar. It serves the purpose of holding both sides of the maxilla stable but also affords us the opportunity to widen the maxilla if needed at the end of the distraction.

The aim of postoperative orthodontic care is to establish a functional occlusion. This work should be timed with the removal of the devices after consolidation. Retention should be planned to make sure the retention appliances are strong. Essex retainers are not typically resistant to the significant transverse pull from the cleft maxilla. Thus, a Hawley retainer or transpalatal support would be better.

## SKELETAL ANCHORS

Regardless of the method of DO (TMDO [Total maxillary DO] or AMD) for the maxilla, the bone has a tendency to move around a point of rotation in the region of the first molar/premolar region in a counterclockwise fashion. Ultimately, as the bone moves forward an open bite will develop unless there is a way to control for this movement and counteract the forces creating this opening. Placing bone anchors/plates in the anterior maxilla and mandible allows placement of interarch elastic traction to prevent this problem. The elastics can also be used during the consolidation phase to maintain the position of the bone.

## THE SURGICAL TECHNIQUE FOR COMPLETE LeFort I DISTRACTION OSTEOGENESIS—INTERNAL AND EXTERNAL DISTRACTORS

Standard LeFort I osteotomy with downfracture is necessary to move the maxilla over long distances. Any sharp projections that may interfere with anterior movement should be removed with rongeurs, or by contouring the bone with a bur. The osteotomy should be made as horizontal as possible to allow for smooth movement forward

**Fig. 9.** VSP of Vector orientation of distractor in the home position.

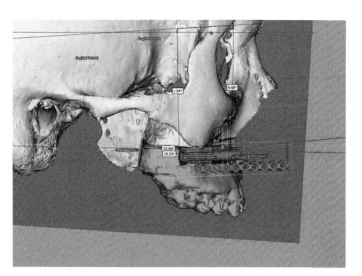

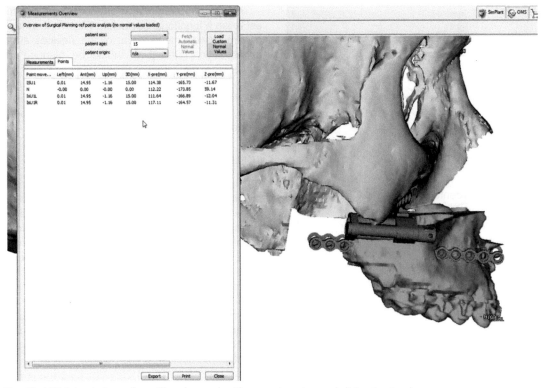

**Fig. 10.** VSP lateral view of maxilla advanced with correct vector and distractor in place.

if that is the vector. Angled osteotomies, if not carefully planned, can lead to obstruction of the maxilla as the bone moves forward. The internal distractors should be aligned and placed before downfracture with the correct vector then removed to allow for downfracture. Once the maxilla is mobilized and down, the maxilla is placed into the correct vector orientation and the

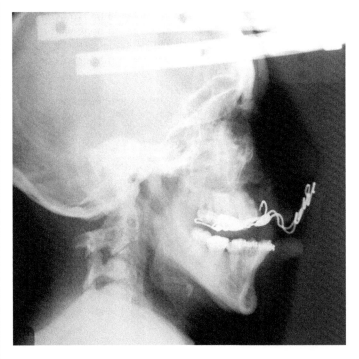

**Fig. 11.** Lateral cephalometric view with RED in place showing attachment to maxilla.

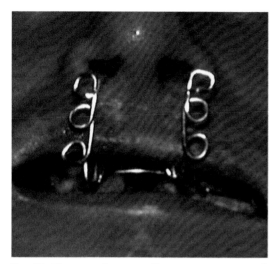

**Fig. 12.** Close up of custom distractor arms to attach to RED external distractor bent to avoid pressure around lips.

devices secured. A suggestion to help obtain a good vector orientation is to use an interocclusal splint, wiring the maxilla to the stable mandible in the vector position that was planned virtually. The vertical position is obtained as the maxilla is brought back up while rotating on the condyles. Placing the devices themselves to the correct vector is also a challenge. Using stereolithic models to prebend the distractors to the vector and then printing device arm orientation devices is quite helpful to improve precision. These arm orientation devices are occlusal based to the maxilla. With small extensions, the distraction pin can be seated to orient the device to the correct vector. Once secured, the devices should be opened to make sure the maxilla will move along its trajectory and then closed back down. The wounds are then closed. The latency period begins.

The external distractors require a separate step after the LeFort downfracture of placing the skull stabilizing halo device to the cranium. This is done after the downfracture. It is positioned such that the vertical arm in the midline, and it is just above the auricles parallel to the horizontal plane. The maxilla appliance is then attached to the vertical arm and the vector adjusted. The wounds are then closed. The vertical arm can be removed for easy extubation then replaced and attached to the devices.

## DEVICE ACTIVATION

A latency of 7 days is recommended to achieve soft callus formation before applying traction across the gap. Variable times have been reported: as soon as 5 days (in younger patients) and up to 7 days, to start turning the distraction rods. The devices should be turned such that only 1 mm per day of activation is achieved.

## CONSOLIDATION

The consolidation period depends on the intramembranous bone calcification along the distraction gap from the periphery to the center. The longer the bone is lengthened, the longer it will take for the fibrous interzone zone to calcify and be strong enough to withstand the forces that may lead to relapse. The most reliable way to know if the bone is hard enough to remove the devices is with a CT scan or cone beam scan looking at the ptyergoid plate region for calcification (**Fig. 13**). However, once the consolidation can be seen clinically along the anterior maxillary wall the distractors can be removed (**Fig. 14**). Once noted, internal devices can be removed. If external distractors are to be used, again, this calcification region also applies. If taken off too soon, even with a face mask traction for stability, there will be some relapse if the bone is too soft. The face mask is not strong enough to withstand the scar tissue and healing of the soft tissues.

The long-term stability has been discussed in studies by Adolph and colleagues, Maazzaini and colleagues, and more recently by Bertrand and colleagues.[20,27,28] The study by Adolph and colleagues suggest that is imperative to allow for complete consolidation of the distraction zone before removing the devices. They advocate for the use of internal devices because these devices are easier to leave in for longer periods to allow for this consolidation to occur. Removing the device too soon could be a possible cause of nonunion of bone associated with external DO in the cleft population. This was further validated by the findings of Bertrand and colleagues. All roads led to the conclusion that taking the devices off too soon could mean a short consolidation time leading to nonunion of bone.

## TOTAL LeFort DISTRACTION VERSUS ANTERIOR MAXILLARY DISTRACTION OSTEOGENESIS IN THE FACE OF VELOPHARYNGEAL INCOMPETENCE

The concept of moving the entire maxilla versus just the anterior alveolus has recently come back into the conversation when planning distraction. Patients who already have VPI or are just on the verge based on testing for this debilitating problem, should be considered for

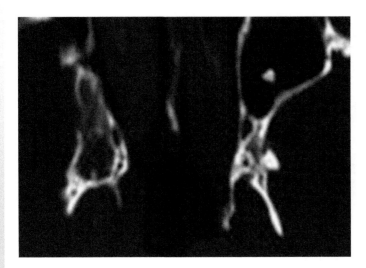

**Fig. 13.** CT confirmation of consolidation at ptyergoid plates.

moving the anterior maxilla only with DO. This leaves the posterior wall of the maxilla in position and does not increase the posterior airway space thus worsening the VPI. Anterior DO also maintains posterior occlusion on the mandibular dentition, preventing supereruption and loss of molar function and occlusion. These osteotomies are created in the bicuspid region. It is necessary to use a combination of distraction devices to control the movement of the vector since it is pulling against the gingival tissues attached to the hard palate. One is placed on the palate, and 2 devices on each side of the maxilla with anchorage against the zygomas or maxillary buttress to push forward. Interarch elastics will also guide the bone and dentition to keep the incisors from rotating superiorly and creating an open bite. Although this may be a bit tricky to learn, it is a reasonable alternative to save the patient from poor molar occlusion and possible VPI.

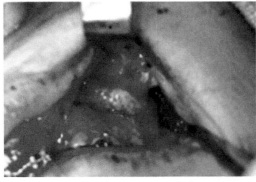

**Fig. 14.** Consolidation of bone across anterior maxilla noted when taking off devices at the end of consolidation.

The development of VPI after total LeFort, whether by DO or conventional osteotomy, has been recognized. The risk factors are difficult to elucidate but are both functional and anatomic in nature.[29] It is known that if the patient has a "borderline" diagnosis of VPI or a short velar length this increases the risk of developing VPI after maxillary advancement by any means.[30] Of note, it is possible to move the entire Lefort without taking down the pharyngeal flap during DO (**Fig. 15**).

## COMPLICATIONS OF LeFort DISTRACTION OSTEOGENESIS

Complications of this process fall into 3 categories: minor, moderate, and severe.[31] As with all surgery there is a risk of swelling, infection, pain, and bleeding. Infection in particular around external pin sites is common. The area of contact between the skull pin and skin appears to be inflamed and colonized with skin flora. The pin sites should appear clean when the pins are removed (**Fig. 16**). Intraorally, the distraction turning rods come through the mucosa and also are colonized by oral flora. These areas need to be kept clean both inside and out. There should be minimal pain with turning the distractor pins, if one encounters severe pain while turning there may be an incomplete osteotomy or premature consolidation of the bone. Bleeding has been reported in the cleft population related to LeFort osteotomy and DO. This is managed the same way as a conventional bleed. Interventional radiology should be used to control the bleeding if direct measures do not work.

Moderate complications are typically related to device issues; the distractor pin loosens, or the distractor rod does not rotate, or the distractor

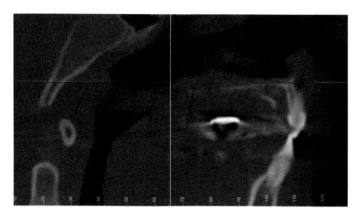

**Fig. 15.** Pharyngeal flap seen on lateral cephalometric view noted to move with DO.

fractures at the solder joints. These usually require replacement of the device. If not replaced the fracture sites are not stable and bone will not consolidate.

Orthodontic complications are related to stability of the appliances placed and the setup of the occlusion if decompensation is needed before surgery. Appliances coming off can lead to lack of transverse stability and loss of control of the distraction process.

Relapse is related to 2 things: taking the distractor off too soon and the bone is not consolidated,[32] the growth of the facial skeleton in a young patient. This should be expected and planned for as best as predictably possible and not treated as relapse.

Severe complications related directly to the DO technique involve the cranial stabilizing pins of the external DO devices inadvertently going through the skull into the brain. This is a neurosurgical emergency and the neurosurgery team should be consulted immediately to help treat this issue.

## SUMMARY

Distraction osteogenesis is a power tool. Although not suggested for most patients requiring orthognathic surgery for cleft skeletal malformations, the technique has been helpful in obtaining stable results for large advancements of the facial skeleton compared with conventional osteotomies. Although strong scientific evidence is sparse, there continue to be many surgeons preferring this technique to conventional osteotomies when challenged with large skeletal movements as noted in the literature.[33,34] More than 5400 articles are listed in PubMed on the topic of DO since the 1970s; however, most are case reports in both the orthopedic and craniofacial literature. Careful patient and case selection is essential to insure adequate compliance and predictability of the process. The use of virtual planning and reverse engineering will enable the orthodontic and surgical team to plan safe and stable surgery. Any surgeon who cares for these special patients should consider incorporating this technique into their armamentarium for difficult cases.

## DISCLOSURE

The authors have nothing to disclose.

## REFERENCES

1. Codavilla A. On the means of lengthening, in the lower limbs, the muscles and tissues which are shortened through deformity. Am J Orthop Surg 1905;(2):353–69.
2. Ilizarov GA. The tension-stress effect on the genesis and growth of tissues. Part I. The influence of stability of fixation and soft-tissue preservation. Clin Orthop Relat Res 1989;(238):249–81.

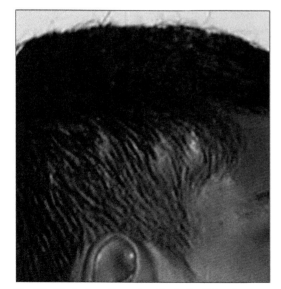

**Fig. 16.** Pin holes after using the halo distractor.

3. Ilizarov GA. The tension-stress effect on the genesis and growth of tissues: Part II. The influence of the rate and frequency of distraction. Clin Orthop Relat Res 1989;(239):263–85.

4. Runyan CM, Gabrick KS. Biology of bone formation, fracture healing, and distraction osteogenesis. J Craniofac Surg 2017;28(5):1380–9.

5. McCarthy JG, Schreiber J, Karp N, et al. Lengthening the human mandible by gradual distraction. Plast Reconstr Surg 1992;89(1):1–8 [discussion: 9–10].

6. Block MS, Brister GD. Use of distraction osteogenesis for maxillary advancement: preliminary results. J Oral Maxillofac Surg 1994;52(3):282–6 [discussion: 287–8].

7. Rachmiel A, Potparic Z, Jackson IT, et al. Midface advancement by gradual distraction. Br J Plast Surg 1993;46(3):201–7.

8. Cohen SR, Corrigan M, Wilmont J, et al. Cumulative operative procedures in patient aged 14 years and older with unilateral or bilateral cleft lip and palate. Plast Reconstr Surg 1995;96(2):267–71.

9. Polley JW, Figueroa AA. Management of severe maxillary deficiency in childhood and adolescence through distraction osteogenesis with an external, adjustable, rigid distraction device. J Craniofac Surg 1997;8(3):181–5 [discussion: 186].

10. Wong GB, Ciminello FS, Padwa BL. Distraction osteogenesis of the cleft maxilla. Facial Plast Surg 2008;24(4):467–72.

11. Le BT, Eyre JM, Wehby MC, et al. Intracranial migration of halo fixation pins: a complication of using an extraoral distraction device. Cleft Palate Craniofac J 2001;38(4):401–4.

12. Brown R, Higuera S, Boyd V, et al. Intracranial migration of a halo pin during distraction osteogenesis for maxillary hypoplasia: a case report and literature review. J Oral Maxillofac Surg 2006;64(1):130–5.

13. Aizenbud D, Rachmiel A, Emodi O. Minimizing pin complications when using the rigid external distraction (RED) system for midface distraction. Oral Surge Oral Med Oral Pathol Oral Radiol Endod 2008;105(2):149–54.

14. Jeblaoui Y, Morand B, Vrix M, et al. maxillary distraction complications in cleft patients. Rev Stomatol Chir Maxillofac 2010;111(3):e1–6.

15. Figueroa AA, Polley JW. Clinical controversies in oral and maxillofacial surgery: part two. External versus internal distraction osteogenesis for the management of severe maxillary hypoplasia: external distraction. J Oral Maxillofac Surg 2008;66(12):2598–604.

16. Drew SJ. Clinical controversies in oral and maxillofacial surgery: Part one. Maxillary distraction osteogenesis for advancement in cleft patients, internal devices. J Oral Maxillofac Surg 2008;66(12):2592–7.

17. Choi C, Park JH, Cha JY, et al. Intraoral premaxillary distraction in a patient with maxillary retrognathic cleft lip and palate: a case report. Cleft Palate Craniofac J 2015;56(6):827–30.

18. Tanikawa C, Lee D, Oonishi YY, et al. The elimination of dental crowding and development of a proper dental arch by maxillary anterior segmental distraction osteogenesis for a patient with UCLP. Cleft Palate Craniofac J 2019;56(7):978–85.

19. Lucchese A, Manuelli M, Albertini P, et al. Treatment of severe maxillary hypoplasia with combined orthodontics and distraction osteogenesis. J Craniofac Surg 2018;29(4):970–2.

20. Adolphs N, Ernst N, Mennekig H, et al. Significance of distraction osteogenesis of the craniomaxillofacial skeleton – a clinical review after 10 years of experience with the technique. J Craniomaxillofac Surg 2014;42:966–75.

21. Liu K, Zhou N. Long-term skeletal changes after maxillary distraction osteogenesis in growing children with cleft lip/palate. J Craniofac Surg 2018;29(4):e349–52.

22. Doucet JC, Herlin C, Gigorre M, et al. Effects of growth on maxillary distraction osteogenesis in cleft lip and palate. J Craniomaxillofac Surg 2013;41(8):836–41.

23. Park YW, Kwon KJ, Kim MK. Long term follow-up of early cleft maxillary distraction. Maxillofac Plast Reconstr Surg 2016;38(1):20.

24. Richardson S, Krishna S, Khandeparker RV. A comprehensive management protocol to treat cleft maxillary hypoplasia. J Craniomaxillofac Surg 2018;46:356–61.

25. Silveria Ad, Moura PM, Harshbarger RJ 3rd. Orthodontic considerations for maxillary distraction osteogenesis in growing patients with cleft lip and palate using internal distractors. Semin Plast Surg 2014;28(4):207–12.

26. Maheshwari S, Verma Sk, Tariq M, et al. Biomechanics and orthodontic treatment protocol in maxillofacial distraction osteogenesis. Natl J Maxillofac Surg 2011;2(2):120–8.

27. Bertrand AA, Lipman KJ, Bradley JP, et al. Consolidation time and relapse: a systematic review of outcomes in internal versus external midface distraction of syndromic craniosynostosis. Plast Reconstr Surg 2019;144(5):1125–34.

28. Maazzaini MD, Basile B, Mazzoleni F, et al. Lonterm follow-up of large maxillary advancements with distraction osteogenesis in growing and non-growing cleft lip and palate patients. J Plast Reconstr Aesthet Surg 2015;68(1):79–86.

29. Vella JB, Tatum SA. Risk factors for velopharyngeal dysfunction following orthognathic suergery in cleft population. Curr Opin Orolaryngol Head Neck Surg 2019;27(4):317–23.

30. McComb RW, Maririnan EM, Nuss RC, et al. Predictors of velopharyngeal insufficiency after Le Fort I maxillary advancement in patients with cleft palate. J Oral Maxillofac Surg 2011;69(8): 2226–32.

31. Moran I, Virdee S, Sharp I, et al. Post-operative complications following Lefort I maxillary surgery in cleft palate patients: a 5 year retrospective study. Cleft Palate Craniofac J 2018;55(2):231–7.

32. He D, Genecov DG, Barcelo R. Nonunion of the external maxillary distraction in cleft lip and palate: analysis of possible reasons. J Oral Maxillofac Surg 2010;68(10):2402–11.

33. Klukos D, Fudalej P, Segueria-byron P, et al. Maxillary distraction osteogenesis versus orthognathic surgery for cleft lip and palate patients. Cochrane Database Syst Rev 2018;(8):CD010403.

34. Austin SL, Mattick CR, Watterhouse PJ. Distraction osteogenesis versus orthognathic surgery for the treatment of maxillary hypoplasia in cleft lip and palate patients: a systematic review. Orthod Craniofac Res 2015;18:96–108.

# Orthodontic and Surgical Principles for Distraction Osteogenesis in Children with Pierre-Robin Sequence

Stephen Yen, DMD, PhD[a,b], Austin Gaal, DDS[c,d], Kevin S. Smith, DDS[c,e,f,g],*

## KEYWORDS

- Mandibular distraction • Pierre-Robin sequence • Tracheostomy • orthodontic
- Temporary anchorage device • Molding of regenerate • Complications • Ankylosis

## KEY POINTS

- Infant mandibular distraction is an effective treatment to improve the airways of patients with Pierre-Robin sequence and can avoid a tracheostomy.
- The management of the distraction procedure is a dynamic process and can be guided with orthodontic support at different stages of distraction and consolidation.
- The orthodontic principles of timing, force, continuous distraction, overcorrection, use of temporary anchorage devices, and balance between stability and molding of the healing callus are described.
- Surgical techniques and complications for mandibular distraction are presented.

## INTRODUCTION: PIERRE-ROBIN SEQUENCE AND DEVELOPMENT OF MANDIBULAR DISTRACTION OSTEOGENESIS

Pierre-Robin sequence (PRS) is seen in infants presenting with the classic triad of glossoptosis, micrognathia, and airway obstruction.[1] A cleft palate may also be seen, but the cleft is not a defining feature of the presentation.[1] The sequence occurs in approximately 1 per 8500 to 1 per 14,000 births; however, there is a disappointing discrepancy among providers in naming the diagnosis and an even greater heterogeneity in treatment protocols.[2] Infants presenting with this triad have a hypoplastic mandible that is retropositioned, allowing the tongue and suprahyoid musculature to impinge and obstruct the airway. The cause of PRS is unknown. Theories include positional malformation in utero, intrinsic mandibular hypoplasia, neurologic/neuromuscular disorders, or a connective tissue disease process.[3]

Historically, the traditional treatment of PRS was tracheostomy, but other potential surgical interventions include tongue lip adhesion (TLA) and mandibular distraction (MDO).[2] TLA involves developing a tongue-genioglossus muscle flap that is anastomosed with the muscle fibers of the orbicularis oris. The tongue heals in this

[a] Division of Dentistry, Children's Hospital Los Angeles, 4650 Sunset Blvd, MS 116, Los Angeles, CA 90027, USA; [b] Center for Craniofacial Molecular Biology, University of Southern California, CSA 103, 2250 Alcazar St. Los Angeles, CA 90033, USA; [c] The University of Oklahoma, College of Dentistry, Department of Oral and Maxillofacial Surgery, JW Keys Cleft and Craniofacial Clinic, 1200 N Stonewall, STE 206, Oklahoma City, OK 73117, USA; [d] Cascadia OMS, 13127 121st Way NE, Kirkland, WA 98034, USA; [e] Children's Hospital of Oklahoma, 1200 Children's Ave Oklahoma City, OK 73104, USA; [f] University of Tulsa, MK Chapman Cleft and Craniofacial Clinic, 2820 East 5th Street, Tulsa, OK 74104, USA; [g] Profiles Oral Facial Surgery Experts, 1000 N Lincoln Blvd, STE 2000, Oklahoma City, OK 73104, USA

* Corresponding author. Profiles Oral Facial Surgery Experts, 1000 N Lincoln Blvd, STE 2000, Oklahoma City, OK 73104.
E-mail address: Kevin-Smith@ouhsc.edu

Oral Maxillofacial Surg Clin N Am 32 (2020) 283–295
https://doi.org/10.1016/j.coms.2020.01.012

advanced position, and it is thought to increase oropharyngeal dimension. Although TLA may seem less invasive compared with MDO and tracheostomy, long-term outcomes are not predictable and the success rate is guarded.[4,5]

In contrast, MDO is established as a reasonable surgical alternative to tracheostomy for these children with congenital mandibular deformities.[6] Although Ilizarov laid the foundations of distraction in the 1960s, it was not until 1992 that McCarthy and colleagues[7] published the use of distraction osteogenesis in the craniofacial skeleton. This technique addresses skeletal deficiencies in mandibular body or ramus length and has been used to rebuild bone in trauma and congenital bony deficiencies in patients with hemifacial microsomia, Treacher Collins syndrome, and PRS. However, distraction osteogenesis is different from orthognathic surgery because the length is obtained by a gradual lengthening of bone that can be difficult to control during the lengthening process; moreover, the final length is prone to relapse unless it is held in position long enough for the bone to mineralize and the soft tissue and muscles to adapt to the new skeletal positions.

This article (1) reviews bone biology related to mandibular distraction, (2) discusses management of mandibular distraction by orthodontic forces, and (3) discusses management of potential complications of distraction osteogenesis.

## BIOLOGY OF DISTRACTION OSTEOGENESIS

In Ilizarov's[8–10] treatise on distraction osteogenesis of the long bones, he divided the distraction procedure into a latency period that was needed for callus formation, a distraction period of active gradual lengthening that determined the length of the bone, and a consolidation period that allowed the stretched callus to mineralize. Usually a cut in the bone is made to create a distraction callus. Then a screw lengthener is attached for gradual lengthening of the callus between the bony segments. The screw lengthener is locked during the consolidation period so that bone can form in the wake of the stretched callus. Ilizarov's[8–10] animal studies suggested that a rate of 1 mm/d was optimal, especially if this 1 mm could be subdivided into multiple smaller increments of lengthening. If the rate was faster, then fibrous union could occur; if slower, then premature consolidation could occur. Stabilization of the segments was essential during the latency period to prevent fibrous union. Once the callus formed, it was possible to distract the callus parallel to the axis of the

long bone, although he showed that it was possible to distract segments in a vector that was perpendicular to the long axis. Ilizarov[8–10] also recommended rigid stabilization during the latency period. The distraction forces on the distraction site caused the callus tissues to reorganize into a fibrous center, a highly vascularized zone of developing bone, and a mineralizing zone of bone undergoing primary bone formation adjacent to the uncut host bone. When tension was applied to move the bony segments apart, mineralization occurred from the bony ends toward the fibrous center.

There are some modifications of the Ilizarov[8–10] prescription when it is applied to the mandible[11]:

1. The latency period can last from 2 days to 1 week following surgery.
2. The mandibular form is not unidirectional. In the past, multidirectional distractors were used to elongate bone along a ramal vertical vector and a body horizontal vector to produce a gonial angle. However, once the distractors were removed, the callus remodeled under the pressure of muscles and soft tissue to produce a smooth curve between the ends of the distractor instead of a gonial angle.
3. Distraction osteogenesis of the ramus tends to place one end of a vertical distractor close to the glenoid fossa, which makes it difficult to remove without an extraoral approach. One solution has been to leave the superior plate of a ramal distractor in the patient after surgery and disengage the rest of the distractor for removal. One difference in planning distraction versus orthognathic surgery is that the screws move to a different position at the end of the distraction and have to be removed. The starting position and the end position of the distractor screws are different so the distractor removal has to be planned at the outset.
4. Age plays an important role in how distractors are placed. During childhood, most of the mandibular bone is filled with developing teeth. It can be difficult to obtain good bony purchase in the ideal preplanned distractor position, which might require placing pins or screws in a nonideal position.
5. During surgery, it is good to test the lengthening of the mandibular distractor by turning the distractor to its end point in order to check for resistance and unexpected forces placed on the distractor. The center of the distraction site is fibrous; therefore, the distraction length can relapse if the bony consolidation is inadequate. Some craniofacial teams overcorrect to

compensate for this potential for relapse. In growing patients, growth predictions based on facial proportions can be used to help estimate how much to lengthen the mandible so that the normally growing midface can catch up to the mandibular position. An antirotation locking pin has been incorporated in the KLS Micro-Zurich distractor used at the University of Oklahoma (OU).

## ANIMAL STUDIES TO DEVELOP ORTHODONTIC PRINCIPLES FOR GUIDING DISTRACTION PROCEDURES

During the 1990s, when mandibular distraction was introduced, there were few guidelines on how to manage mandibular distraction when side effects developed, such as the development of open bites or mandibular deviation during the distraction process. The laboratory at the Center for Craniofacial Molecular Biology at University of Southern California (USC) recreated problems encountered in mandibular distraction using a rabbit animal model.[12–14] The group then tested how the side effects developed and how orthodontic forces could be used to correct them.

It was noted that, if the distractors were not placed parallel to the occlusal plane, then horizontal lengthening did not occur; instead, the mandible could develop an open bite because of a downward positioning of the distractor. To simulate what would happen if screws loosened during distraction, Yen and colleagues[13] tested what would happen if stable distractor pins were pitted against unstable pins. This procedure was performed by reducing the number of stable screws on one side of a bilateral mandibular distraction procedure. When 4 pins were pitted against 3, or 3 against 2, the mandible deviated to the less stable side without an open bite even if the distractors were placed in a downward position. Four distractor screws, two per segment, was the minimum number of for the segments to elongate along the axis of the distractor. If fewer than 2 screws were used to simulate loosening of 1 screw, then the segments tended to rotate if the distractors were placed 35° downward from the occlusal plane. Rather than create an open bite like a stable distractor, the distractors produced a rotation of the anterior segment to close the bite with a hinge-like movement. Once rotational movements could be planned by offsetting the distractors and placed using only 1 screw in each segment, then it was possible to reproducibly create 8-mm to 12-mm anterior open bites because of mandibular segmental rotations. These open

bites were enormous relative to the size of the animal. The research question then evolved into how to close the open bites with orthodontic forces.

To test how orthodontic elastics or springs could be used to guide a mandibular distraction procedure, researchers at USC examined the response in 100 rabbits when the forces and timing of spring applications were different. From these studies, several principles emerged:

1. If the elastics were added after 2 months of consolidation, heavy elastic forces could not close an iatrogenic open bite created during the mandibular distraction procedure. The bone had consolidated and resisted attempts to mold the callus. If forces were placed on the teeth, then the teeth extruded under pressure.

2. It was possible to close an open bite and mold the distraction callus during distraction and the first 2 weeks of consolidation period with heavy elastic forces. Light elastic forces could not overpower the distractors. Whenever possible, temporary anchorage device (TAD) or intermaxillary fixation screws should be placed in the bone. A wire loop should be connected from the TAD to the archwire so that interarch elastics placed on the archwire transmit the forces to the TAD and prevent extrusion of teeth.

3. During distraction and the first 2 weeks of consolidation, it was possible to obtain correction of open bites created during the distraction process. If elastics were used later, only partial correction was attained. Other centers, such as OU, have also encountered open bites; however, those cases closed without using elastics.

4. Once distraction was started, it had to be continued until the desired length was obtained. If the patient stopped the distraction procedure by forgetting to turn the distraction screw, then a paper-thin cortical plate rapidly enveloped the distraction site and stopped the distraction process. A scalpel was required to slice this thin layer if the distraction process was restarted. In the rabbit, this layer was visualized on micro-computed tomography imaging 3 days after the distraction stopped. Bone could be seen in the distraction site after 2 to 3 weeks of distraction because the bone was placed under tension.

5. The center of the distraction site was fibrous and could be stretched during the distraction stage to produce bone so that bone mineralized from the ends toward the fibrous center. When the distractors were removed early, the fibrous center could cause relapse.

Overcorrection is recommended for distraction procedures to compensate for postsurgical relapse.

6. Hoffmeister and colleagues[15] presented the floating bone concept: distractors are removed after 2 weeks of consolidation so that the distraction callus can be molded with elastic forces in order to improve the occlusion. In the rabbit, if the distractors were removed earlier than 2 weeks, the elastic forces caused the unsupported distraction site to buckle toward the less stable side and caused bending of the mandible. The 2 weeks of consolidation allowed the thin cortical plates to give the distraction site some lateral stability. Therefore, vertical elastics would not cause buckling of the distraction site.

7. If elastics are applied during the distraction procedure or during the first 2 weeks of consolidation, it is recommended that the distractors be left in place while applying guiding elastics. If the distractors are removed and the elastics are applied, then this should be done 2 weeks after distraction has stopped.

The following cases (**Figs. 1** and **2**) show how mandibular distraction is used at CHLA in infants with mandibular retrognathia and respiratory distress in order to avoid a tracheostomy.[16,17] At CHLA, many newborns have required a tracheostomy. The center at CHLA has followed more than 70 patients using this distraction protocol. With time, the gonial angle tended to open with infant distraction (**Fig. 1**B).

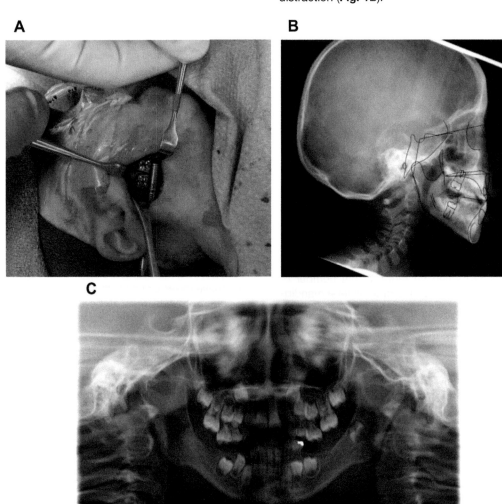

**Fig. 1.** (*A*) Inverted-L osteotomy for infant mandibular distraction to treat respiratory distress and retrognathic mandible as described by Urata and Hammoudeh[33] at Children's Hospital Los Angeles. (*B*) Cephalometric radiograph shows normal profile despite liner gonial angle (*C*) panoramic radiograph shows missing molar teeth in older patients who underwent infant mandibular distraction. Facial profile looks normal.

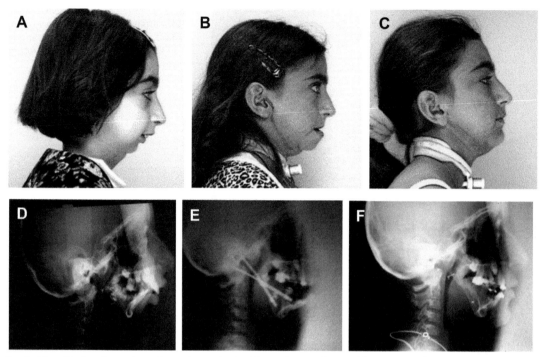

**Fig. 2.** Mandibular distraction of a patient who had 2 previous orthognathic surgeries. (*A, D*) Presurgical records in May. (*B, E*) Distraction alone with an offset position of the distractors in June. (*C, F*) After orthodontic guidance in September. (*From* Yen SL, Gross J,Yamashita DD, et al. Correcting an anterior open-bite side effect during distraction with spring forces. Plast Reconstr Surg. 2002;110(6):1482; with permission.)

The second example shows how the limitations of the mandibular distraction vector can be improved with orthodontic guidance.[18] This patient was flown from Russia, where she had multiple mandibular surgeries, all unsuccessful because of surgical site infections. When the patient was brought to CHLA, the same strategy was not used because it already failed twice. A distraction vector was planned that would provide horizontal lengthening; however, the surgeons had to try out different screw positions because they could not achieve good bony purchase in the ideal position. The position that allowed screw placement resembled the position the research group at CCMB had seen before in rabbit experiments that created an open bite. **Fig. 2** shows the patient at the end of distraction. By taking baseline films at the beginning and progress films, the group could reconstruct the direction and path of mandibular lengthening. The anterior segment rotated inferiorly because of the offset position of the distractors. To correct it, counter-rotation was used with class III elastics and anterior vertical elastics. **Fig. 2**C shows the orthodontic correction of the mandibular distal segment and a pleasing surgical and orthodontic outcome of the procedure.

## MANDIBULAR DISTRACTION SURGICAL TECHNIQUE USED AT UNIVERSITY OF OKLAHOMA

Buschman and Smith[19] reported in 2000 at the American Cleft Palate-Craniofacial Association Annual Meeting one of the earliest series of mandibular distraction for neonatal obstructive sleep apnea. Another of the earliest reported series of internal mandibular distraction was by Smith[20] in 2001, at the 3rd International Congress on Cranial and Facial Bone Distraction Processes. He described his experience with 5 neonates (mean age, 31 days) with a mean follow-up of 10 months. All patients were weaned from intubation on the completion of distraction consolidation, and those neonates who had preoperative sleep studies showed a mean reduction in Apnea-Hypopnea Index (AHI) by 44%.[20]

Along with the expanding literature on mandibular distraction osteogenesis (MDO) outcomes, there are multiple technical variations to achieve the end goal. The following is a brief description of the technique followed at the institution at OU[20–22]:

1. Intubation. Oral, nasal, or tracheostomy may be used, but the endotracheal tube must be managed and positioned out of the surgical field.

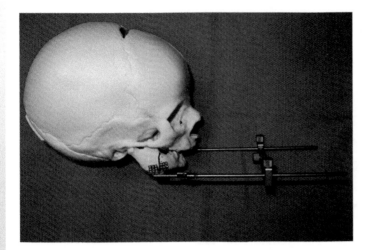

**Fig. 3.** Distractor used at OU along with paralleling guide. (*Courtesy of* Austin J. Gaal, DDS, and Kevin S. Smith, DDS, Oral and Maxillofacial Surgery, University of Oklahoma, 2019.)

2. Access to posterior mandibular body and ramus by transcervical approach. Trauma to the marginal mandibular branch is a well-known anatomic consideration. Because these infants have a limited volume status, the risk for transfusion requirement and major complications (hemorrhage, stroke, myocardial infarct) is heightened to a much greater degree.

3. Try on distractor. The team at OU uses the KLS Micro-Zurich distractor, which needs to be adapted to the mandible in the site where the anticipated osteotomy is to be performed. The curvature of the mandible in the axial plane must be considered. The goal is to distract the distal segment of the mandible forward, parallel to the midsagittal plane. Therefore, the distractor plates must be accurately adapted to follow the convexity and curve of the lateral ramus/posterior body. A paralleling guide (available from KLS-Martin) may be used to verify vector direction (**Fig. 3**).

4. The contralateral access, distractor adaptation, and corticotomy must be performed so that the distractor arms are parallel in vector. Adjustments in angulation may be necessary and should be done before both corticotomies are completed.

5. Perform corticotomy in an inverted-L configuration. A 701 fissure bur is used, and corticotomy is made only through the buccal cortex, being careful not to violate tooth buds (**Fig. 4**).

6. The activation arm protrudes near the area of the parasymphysis. An additional stab incision is necessary for the arm to exit the skin. The activation arm may exit anteriorly or posteriorly, but the craniofacial team at OU favors the arm exiting anteriorly. The group has

experienced some children developing skin ulceration near their mastoids if the arm exits posteriorly.

7. Fixate the distractor to the mandible. At least 3 screws on either side of the corticotomy must stabilize the hardware (**Fig. 5**).

8. Activate the distractor to confirm that separation between mandibular proximal and distal segments has been completed. Turn the activation arm multiple times such that an advancement of at least 1 cm is visualized to confirm that no greenstick fracture will occur inadvertently while the child is undergoing distraction.

9. Return the distractor back to its preactivated arm's length. The distractor used at OU incorporates an antirotation locking pin, which must be switched to the proper configuration (**Fig. 6**).

10. Wound toilet and closure.

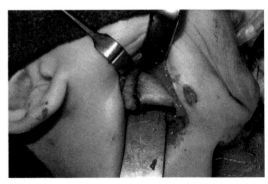

**Fig. 4.** Inverted-L corticotomy used by the center at OU. (*Courtesy of* Austin J. Gaal, DDS, and Kevin S. Smith, DDS, Oral and Maxillofacial Surgery, University of Oklahoma, 2019.)

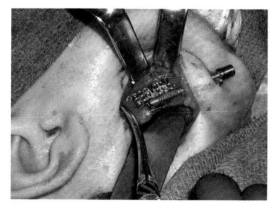

**Fig. 5.** Distractor adapted and fixated in place. (*Courtesy of* Austin J. Gaal, DDS, and Kevin S. Smith, DDS, Oral and Maxillofacial Surgery, University of Oklahoma, 2019.)

## COMPLICATIONS

As suggested by the review on the mandibular distraction technique, MDO may result in several complications. Although there is an expanding volume of literature supporting the success of MDO and the ability to keep children from requiring a tracheostomy, clinicians must be cognizant of these potential issues that may arise.[6,23,24] Only now are longer-term studies becoming available. Even less literature is available that is specific to patients with PRS.[25,26] Therefore, there is no standard classification system for the complications

of MDO. For the sake of simplicity, complications are discussed here in relation to early and late subsets.

### Early

Early complications of MDO include perioperative, intraoperative, and postoperative encounters, which include major anesthetic catastrophes such as hemorrhage, shock, and death. These catastrophes are rare, so far, in the MDO experience. However, they do occur on occasion and are reported in the literature from centers with robust patient volumes. For example, the Royal Children's Hospital recently audited their experience retrospectively on 73 children with MDO.[27] Both syndromic and nonsyndromic cases were included, and the average patient age at the time of MDO was 2 to 3 months.[27] Out of 73 cases, 2 infants died at home after distraction. One infant with Toriello-Carey syndrome aspirated and had respiratory arrest during sleep, which was before distractor removal.[27] The second child (Treacher Collins syndrome) died 2 years after distractor removal and during a failed tracheostomy tube change.[27] In another report of 50 patients with MDO, there was 1 death, a cardiopulmonary event that occurred 32 months after distractor removal.[28] The patient had a preexisting ventricular septal defect, pulmonary hypertension, right ventricular hypertrophy, and laryngomalacia.[28] Murage and colleagues[28] also reported on pooled

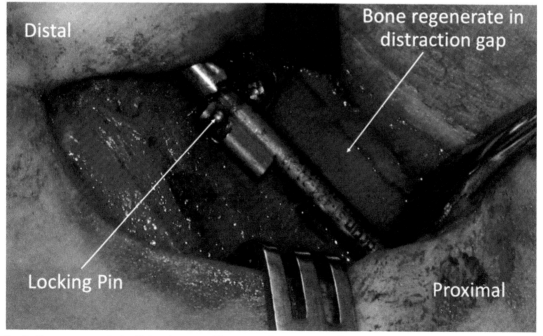

**Fig. 6.** Bone regenerate in distraction gap. (*Courtesy of* Austin J. Gaal, DDS, and Kevin S. Smith, DDS, Oral and Maxillofacial Surgery, University of Oklahoma, 2019.)

**Table 1**
Comparison of studies reporting complications of mandibular distraction in patients with Robin sequence

| Studies | | | | Complications | | | |
| --- | --- | --- | --- | --- | --- | --- | --- |
| Author, Year | n | Placement | Type of Distractor | Total | Major | Moderate | Minor |
| Murage et al,[30] 2013 | 50 | Internal | Nonresorbable | 30% | 0% | 12% SSI (10%) Device fracture requiring repeat distraction (2%) | 18% SSI (12%) Facial neuropraxia (2%) Self-extubation (4%) |
| Andrews et al,[31] 2013 | 73 | Internal | Nonresorbable | 29% | 16% Dental injury (6%) TMJ ankylosis (10%) | Widened neck scars (8%) | SSI (5%) |
| Breugem et al,[33] 2012 | 12 | Internal | Resorbable | 17% | — | Extrusion of distraction screw (8%) | SSI (8%) |
| Hammoudeh et al,[16] 2012 | 29 | Internal | Nonresorbable | 18% | Death 3.4% (n = 1) | 6.80% Device failure requiring replacement 3.4% (n = 1) Exposure of distraction device 3.4% (n = 1) | 6.80% Facial nerve palsy 3.4% (n = 1) SSI 3.4% (n = 1) |
| Hong et al,[32] 2012 | 6 | Internal | Nonresorbable | 33% | — | — | SSI (n = 1) |
| Zenha et al, 2012 | 2 | Internal | Nonresorbable | 50% | — | — | Delay in distractor removal (n = 1) |
| Allam et al,[27] 2011 | 9 | Internal | Nonresorbable | 33% | 0% | 22% Abscess requiring incision and drainage (n = 2) | 11% Facial nerve palsy (n = 1) |
| Mahirous Mohamed et al, 2011 | 11 | Internal | Nonresorbable | 45% | — | 36% Incomplete osteotomy (n = 1) SSI (n = 3) | 9% Facial nerve palsy (n = 1) |
| Scott et al, 2011 | 19 | External | Nonresorbable | 84% | 26.30% Dental injury 21% (n = 4) Residual anterior open bite 5.3% (n = 1) | — | Hypertrophic scars (15.8%. n = 3) Facial nerve injury (15.8%. n = 3) SSI (26.3%. n = 5) |

| Study | n | Device | Fixation | | Bilateral odontomas | | |
|---|---|---|---|---|---|---|---|
| Hammoudeh et al, 2009 | 1 | External | Nonresorbable | NA | — | — | — |
| Genecov et al, 2009 | 67 | Both | Both | 35.4% | Device failure requiring replacement (13.2%) | 22.20% | SSI (13.3%) Transient facial neuropraxia (8.9%) |
| | | Internal (49%) | — | — | — | | SSI (13.3%) |
| | | | Resorbable lateral screws | — | 3% | 4.5% | 4.45% |
| | | External (51%) | Nonresorbable | — | 10.20% | | 8.8%, 4.45% |
| Burstein and Williams, 2005 | 15 | Internal | Resorbable | — | — | SSI (26.7%) | |
| Denny and Kalantanan, 2002 | 5 | External | Nonresorbable | 20 | — | Early distractor removal (n = 1) | |
| Monasterio et al, 2002 | 15 | External | Nonresorbable | 20 | — | 20% SSI (n = 1) Pin loosening (n = 2) | |

**Average Complication Rates**

| Total No. of Patients = 337 | Total (%) | Major (%) | Moderate (%) | Minor (%) |
|---|---|---|---|---|
| — | 34 | 9 | 15.10 | 15 |

n indicates number of patients in the study who underwent distraction osteogenesis.

*Abbreviation:* SSI, surgical site infection.

*From* Murage KP, Costa MA, Friel MT, et al. Complications associated with neonatal mandibular distraction osteogenesis in the treatment of Robin sequence. J Craniofac Surg. 2014;25:385; with permission.

MDO complications, cited from several earlier studies, from 2002 to 2013 (**Table 1**).

Surgical complications include anatomic, technical misadventures with the corticotomy, and distractor malfunction. Early in the postoperative period, infections, hardware exposure, dental trauma, distraction vector issues, premature consolidation of the regenerate, device failure, hypertrophic scarring, and asymmetry may be noted.[3,26] Out of 35 patients with MDO (extraoral technique), the most common complication was development of an anterior open bite.[3] Guiding elastics have not been necessary to mold the regenerate at OU, although they may be a consideration for practitioners, as described from the CHLA group. Miloro[3] reported that all anterior open bites resolved on their own within 3 months following device removal.

Infections may be minor, warranting a brief antibiotic course, or they may become major and require return to the operative room. According to a recent single-center 7-year retrospective review of 50 patients with MDO, the most common complication was infection, with an alarming rate of 22%.[28] Most cases resolved with antibiotics alone and did not require reoperation.[28] The question then is whether there is an overdiagnosis of infection and resultant overprescription of antibiotics. It has been the experience at OU that most patients with MDO present with chronic erythema and drainage around the site of the distract arms. The erythema may last during the entire distraction and consolidation periods. Adhikari and colleagues[27] reported this finding in 41% of patients. The erythema and drainage resolve after device removal at the end of consolidation.

The question of whether to use an internal or external distractor may affect the likelihood of hypertrophic scarring, hardware failure, and need for reoperation. Although Miloro[3] reported a favorable experience with his external distractors, other studies support the use of internal distractors. Paes and colleagues[29] conducted a systematic review of 12 studies comparing the outcomes of patients treated with internal versus external distractors, and better outcomes and fewer complications were associated with internal distractors. A more recent (2016) review of 43 studies agrees with Paes and colleagues[29] that there are higher rates of complications and risk of scarring when using external distractors.[23]

Surgical failure may be defined as any cause for early reoperation.[23] Reasons for surgical failure may be multifactorial, and the primary cause may be difficult to pinpoint. Several reasons for surgical failure are listed in **Table 2**.[23]

**Table 2**
**Reported reasons for surgical failure**

| Reason for Failure | No. of Patients |
|---|---|
| Incomplete osteotomy | 1 |
| Premature consolidation | 1 |
| Pin dislodgement | 3 |
| Device failure | 2 |
| Exposure of distractor | 1 |
| Nonunion | 1 |
| Coronoid ankylosis | 1 |
| Mandibular fracture | 1 |
| No details provided | 8 |

*From* Breik O, Tivey D, Umapathysivam K, et al. Does the rate of distraction or type of distractor affect the outcome of mandibular distraction in children with micrognathia? J Oral Maxillofac Surg. 2016;74:1447; with permission.

### Late

Some complications take many years to come to fruition, especially with trauma to molar tooth buds. In a retrospective review of 26 patients who underwent mandibular distraction, greater than 1-year follow-up on these children confirmed that more than 85% of patients experienced adverse effects to dental buds.[26] This review was from a single institution and the average patient age during time of MDO was 8 years old.[26] However, infants with PRS undergoing distraction are usually managed with this treatment earlier in life. In a retrospective cohort study from the Netherlands, the average patient age during MDO was 3.7 months.[30] The investigators compared 10 patients with PRS undergoing MDO with 10 patients with PRS who did not undergo MDO with at least 5-year follow-up. Dental shape anomalies, positional changes, and molar root malformations were significantly increased in the MDO group compared with the control group.[30] In 1 study, investigators recommended prophylactic removal of molar follicles at the site of osteotomy with hopes to improve bone formation at the distraction site.[31]

Failure to relieve the airway obstruction or decannulate may present any time during the patient's early life.[3] Out of 8 tracheostomy-dependent patients undergoing MDO, 2 patients were not decannulated.[27] Out of a different group's 50 patients with MDO, 4 patients required a tracheostomy following distraction.[28]

An especially ominous complication, temporomandibular joint (TMJ) ankylosis, may not present for several years after MDO. One case of TMJ ankylosis has been experienced at OU (**Fig. 7**).

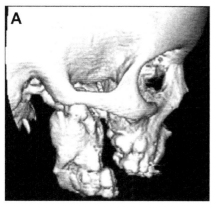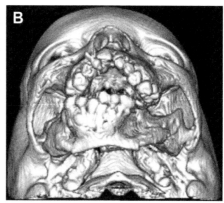

**Fig. 7.** (*A,B*) Patient that had had multiple mandiblar distractions at another institution seen for consult to correct severe mandibular ankylosis. (*Courtesy of* Austin J. Gaal, DDS, and Kevin S. Smith, DDS, Oral and Maxillofacial Surgery, University of Oklahoma, 2019.)

The Royal Children's Hospital also reported 1 case of TMJ ankylosis.[27] The coronoid has been described to fuse with the posterior maxilla in another MDO complication.[23] However, the inverted-L design in that report incorporated the coronoid process in the distal mandibular segment. At OU, the corticotomy design keeps the coronoid process in the proximal segment of the mandible (see **Figs. 3** and **4**).

## REQUIRING ADDITIONAL PROCEDURES

In addition, the question of whether MDO causes growth disturbance is just now beginning to be answered. In 2 retrospective studies, mandibular growth of children with MDO was analyzed with a mean follow-up of 4 to 5 years.[26,29] Both studies suggest that the mandibles of children with MDO remain shorter and do not catch up in growth compared with children who did not undergo distraction.[26,29] This finding may necessitate further procedures (ie, mandibular sagittal split osteotomy) on the completion of somatic growth, which is exactly what was forecasted by Shand and colleagues[22] during distraction's introduction in 2004.[29] The following conclusions have been made from long-term follow-up on several patients treated at OU:

1. MDO offers a tool to significantly, although less accurately, advance the mandible when indicated.
2. Definitive orthognathic surgery is usually indicated at the completion of growth in order to fine tune the mandible's final position and occlusion.
3. MDO is indicated if a neonate otherwise would require a tracheostomy. MDO offers a safer long-term alternative and quality of life, thus

the need to perform orthognathic surgery is not considered a complication of MDO.

It is critical to appropriately select the patients who would benefit most from MDO. In an effort to improve patient selection, Flores and colleagues[6] (2015) developed the GIANTO [GER (gastroesophageal reflux), age >30, neurologic anomaly, airway anomalies other than laryngomalacia, intact palate, and preoperative intubation] score in a single-center study to accurately predict which patients would fail MDO. Miloro[3] suggested a more clinician-based assessment. His indications for MDO include micrognathia with a maxillomandibular discrepancy or overjet of more than −8 mm, repetitive upper airway symptoms with chronic low $Spo_2$ readings, repeat apnea monitor triggering, labored breathing or cyanosis, poor oral intake, lack of weight gain consistent with age, or abnormal sleep studies as long as central apnea has been ruled out.[3] Laryngoscopy showing

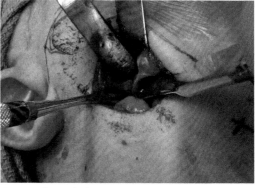

**Fig. 8.** Aborted distraction. (*Courtesy of* Austin J. Gaal, DDS, and Kevin S. Smith, DDS, Oral and Maxillofacial Surgery, University of Oklahoma, 2019.)

obstruction at tongue base without significant laryngomalacia or tracheomalacia is the next step in diagnosis.[3] Patients who are not MDO candidates are those with mild airway compromise controlled by positional maneuvers, central apnea, secondary airway lesions (tracheomalacia), or a floppy epiglottis.[3]

## SUMMARY

Mandibular distraction has continued to gain popularity, with other surgeons such as Denny and colleagues,[24] Sidman, Chigurapati, and Monasterio reporting outcomes.[21,34–36] In a comprehensive literature review (1981–2015), only 3 out of 84 patients with distraction had persistent obstruction defined by severe AHI on polysomnography (PSG), giving a success rate of 96%.[6] In Breik and colleagues'[23] systematic review of 43 studies, the overall success of MDO was 95.4%.

However, there remains heterogeneity among surgical providers in providing care for infants with PRS. In a recent survey sent to surgeons of the American Cleft Palate-Craniofacial Association, only 48% of respondents preferred to manage the airway with distraction.[2] These surgeons included oral and maxillofacial surgeons, plastics surgeons, and otolaryngologists. Perhaps the treatment modality of choice depends more on the training and background of the surgeon than on objective data. In orthopedic surgery, there is a learning curve that describes the stabilization of complications with experience.[32] This learning curve can also apply to the craniofacial teams learning to manage mandibular distraction. There can be initial enthusiasm about distraction's potential, then a dampening of this enthusiasm as complications appear with larger numbers of trials.

In summary, MDO is a powerful tissue engineering technique for generating additional bone in patients with bony deficiency, but it is difficult to teach distraction osteogenesis to residents who have not experienced the learning curve. It is not to be attempted without an experienced surgeon and orthodontist present, because this could be a recipe for disaster, producing the complications rather than the desired mandibular lengthening. Experience shows that there are cases in which MDO does not work **(Fig. 8)**. However, in many cases of severe retrognathia, MDO has saved patients from a tracheostomy. MDO is not as accurate as orthognathic surgery, and secondary procedures are usually indicated at the completion of growth. In experienced hands, MDO is predictable and reproducible, with success rates more than 95%, defined by PSG. In the future, with increasingly objective and pooled outcome data, it is hoped that appropriate patient and treatment selection will be optimized using a team approach.

## ACKNOWLEDGMENTS

The distraction strategies were developed from research studies support by the American Association of Oral and Maxillofacial Surgeons, the American Association of Orthodontists Foundation and the Chalmer J. Lyons Academy.

## DISCLOSURE

K. S. Smith receives royalty from KLS-Martin for product development, no other conflicts.

## REFERENCES

1. Robin P. Glossoptosis due to atresia and hypotrophy of the mandible. Am J Dis Child 1934;48:541–7.
2. Collins B. Airway management in Pierre Robin sequence: patterns of practice. Cleft Palate Craniofac 2014;51(3):283–9.
3. Miloro M. Mandibular distraction Osteogenesis for pediatric airway management. J Oral Maxillofac Surg 2010;68:1512–23.
4. Menashe VD, Farrehi C, Miller M. Hypoventilation and cor pulmonale due to chronic upper airway obstruction. J Pediatr 1965;67:198.
5. Resnick CM, Calabrese CE, Sahdev R, et al. Is tongue-lip adhesion or mandibular distraction more effective in relieving obstructive apnea in infants with robin sequence? J Oral Maxillofac Surg 2019; 77:591–600.
6. Flores RL, Greathouse ST, Costa M, et al. Defining failure and its predictors in mandibular distraction for Robin sequence. J Craniomaxillofac Surg 2015; 43:1614–9.
7. McCarthy JG, Schreiber J, Karp N, et al. Lengthening the human mandible by gradual distraction. Plast Reconstr Surg 1992;89(1).
8. Ilizarov GA. The tension-stress effect on the genesis and growth of tissues: II. The influence of the rate and frequency on distraction. Clin Orthop 1989; 239:263–85.
9. Ilizarov GA. The tension-stress effect on the genesis and growth of tissues: I. The influence of stability on fixation and soft-tissue preservation. Clin Orthop 1989;238:249–81.
10. Ilizarov GA. The principles of the Ilizarov method. Bull Hosp Jt Dis Orthop Inst 1988;48:1–18.
11. Yen SL. Distraction osteogenesis: application to dentofacial orthopedics. Semin Orthod 1997;3: 275–83.
12. Yen SL, Shang W, Shuler C, et al. Orthodontic spring guidance of bilateral mandibular distraction in

rabbits. Am J Orthod Dentofacial Orthop 2001;120: 435–42.

13. Yen SL, Wei S, Shuler C, et al. Bending of the distraction site during mandibular distraction osteogenesis in the rabbit: a model for studying segment control and side effects. J Oral Maxillofac Surg 2001;59:779–88.

14. Wei S, Scadeng M, Yamashita DD, et al. Manipulating the distraction site at different stages of consolidation. J Oral Maxillofac Surg 2007;65: 840–6.

15. Hoffmeister B, Marks C, Wolff K. Floating bone concept in mandibular distraction. Int J Oral Maxillofac Surg 1999;28:90.

16. Hammoudeh J, Bindingnavele VK, Davis B, et al. Neonatal and infant mandibular distraction as an alternative to tracheostomy in severe obstructive sleep apnea. Cleft Palate Craniofac J 2012;49(1): 32–8.

17. Mobin SS, Francis CS, Karatsonyi AL, et al. Mandibular distraction instead of tracheostomy in Pierre Robin sequence patients: is it worth it? Plast Reconstr Surg 2012;130(5):766e–7e.

18. Yen SL, Gross J, Yamashita DD, et al. Correcting an anterior open bite side effect during distraction with spring forces. Plast Reconstr Surg 2002;110: 1476–84.

19. Buschman J, Smith K. Treatment of obstructive sleep apnea with distraction osteogenesis. 57th Annual Meeting and Pre-Conference Symposium: Distraction Osteogenesis in the Facial Skeleton. American Cleft Palate- Craniofacial Association. Atlanta, Apr 10-15, 2000.

20. Smith KS. Internal distraction in neonates, treatment of obstructive apnea. 3rd International Congress on Cranial and Facial Bone Distraction Processes: 2001 Distraction Odyssey. Monduzzi Editore, Medimond. Paris, June14-16, 2001.

21. Shand JM. Mandibular distraction in infancy for airway obstruction. Atlas of oral and maxillofacial surgery. St Louis (MO): Elsevier; 2015.

22. Shand JM, Smith KS, Heggie AA. The role of distraction osteogenesis in the management of craniofacial syndromes. Oral Maxillofacial Surg Clin North Am 2004;16:525–40.

23. Breik O, Tivey D, Umapathysivam K, et al. Does the rate of distraction or type of distractor affect the outcome of mandibular distraction in children with micrognathia? J Oral Maxillofac Surg 2016;74: 1441–53.

24. Denny A, Kalantarian B. Mandibular distraction in neonates: a strategy to avoid tracheostomy. Plast Reconstr Surg 2002;109:896–904.

25. Zhang RS, Lin LO, Hoppe IC, et al. Early mandibular distraction in craniofacial microsomia and need for orthognathic correction at skeletal maturity: a comparative long-term follow-up study. Plast Reconstr Surg 2018;142:1285.

26. Peacock ZS, Salcines A, Troulis MJ, et al. Long-term effects of distraction osteogenesis of the mandible. J Oral Maxillofac Surg 2018;76:1512–23.

27. Adhikari AN, Heggie AA, Shand JM, et al. Infant mandibular distraction for upper airway obstruction: a clinical audit. Plast Reconstr Surg Glob Open 2016;4:e812.

28. Murage KP, Costa MA, Friel MT, et al. Complications Associated with neonatal mandibular distraction osteogenesis in the treatment of robin sequence. J Craniofac Surg 2014;25:383–7.

29. Paes EC, Mink van der Molen AB, Muradin MS, et al. A systematic review on the outcome of mandibular distraction osteogenesis in infants suffering Robin sequence. Clin Oral Investig 2013;17:8.

30. Paes EC, Bittermann GK, Bittermann D, et al. Long-term results of mandibular distraction osteogenesis with a resorbable device in infants with robin sequence: effects on developing molars and mandibular growth. Plast Reconstr Surg 2016;137: 375e.

31. Regev E, Jensen JN, McCarthy JG, et al. Removal of mandibular tooth follicles before distraction osteogenesis. Plast Reconstr Surg 2004;113:1910.

32. Dahl MT, Gulli B, Berg T. Complications of limb lengthening. A learning curve. Clin Orthop 1994; 301:10–8.

33. Hammoudeh JA, Fahradyan A, Brady C, et al. Predictors of failure in infant mandibular distraction osteogenesis. J Oral Maxillofac Surg 2018;76(9): 1955–65.

34. Sidman JD, Sampson D, Templeton B. Distraction osteogenesis of the mandible for airway obstruction in children. Laryngoscope 2001;111:1137.

35. Chigurupati R, Massie J, Dargaville P, et al. Internal mandibular distraction to relieve airway obstruction in infants and young children with micrognathia. Pediatr Pulmonol 2004;37:230.

36. Monasterio FO, Drucker M, Molina F, et al. Distraction osteogenesis in Pierre Robin sequence and related respiratory problems in children. J Craniofac Surg 2002;13:79.

# Orthodontics for Unilateral and Bilateral Cleft Deformities

Yassmin Parsaei, DMD[a], Flavio Uribe, DDS, MDentSc[a],*,
Derek Steinbacher, MD, DMD[b]

## KEYWORDS

- Cleft orthodontics • Cleft orthopedics • Bilateral cleft lip and palate • Unilateral cleft lip and palate

## KEY POINTS

- Understands the common dentofacial abnormalities present in UCLP and BCLP patients.
- Describes orthodontic, orthopedic, and surgical treatment modalities for the cleft patient.
- Provides a brief review of the literature illustrating the use and efficacy of the various treatment approaches.

## INTRODUCTION

Patients with unilateral or bilateral cleft lip and palate (UCLP and BCLP) require extensive orthodontic treatment in an effort to achieve optimal dental occlusion and orofacial esthetics. Such patients often present with dental and esthetic impairments including midface deficiencies, dental crossbites, dental anomalies, asymmetries of the soft tissues, and extraoral and intraoral soft-tissue scarring, as well as feeding and speech difficulties. A multidisciplinary approach is therefore essential in achieving optimal treatment outcomes.

The role of the orthodontist is central in the overall management of patients with unilateral and bilateral cleft deformities. Orthodontic treatment may be performed at different stages of development and can vary depending on severity of the cleft, amount of jaw discrepancy, and the presence of dental abnormalities. Although clefts of the lip may require limited or no orthodontic treatment, severe types affecting the lip, alveolar process, and palate (UCLP or BCLP) often require more complex management strategies. Active phases of treatment may be divided into the following stages:

1. Orthodontic-orthopedic treatment in the early mixed dentition
2. Orthodontic-orthopedic treatment in the late mixed dentition
3. Orthodontic treatment/surgical preparation in the adult dentition

Following lip and palatal closure at 3 and 12 months, respectively, maxillary growth is often diminished in the vertical, sagittal, and transverse planes. Orthodontic-orthopedic treatment aims to improve midfacial growth and correct anterior and posterior dental crossbites. As permanent teeth erupt, dental anomalies in the cleft patient, such as missing, supernumerary, and dislocated teeth, have a large influence on the orthodontic treatment plan. As the transverse dimension is addressed, securing the eruption of teeth with normal morphology into the arch is of primary importance.

It is important to make note of the use of presurgical orthopedics and nasoalveolar molding,

[a] Division of Orthodontics, Department of Craniofacial Sciences, University of Connecticut, 263 Farmington Avenue, Farmington, CT 06032, USA; [b] Section of Plastic and Reconstructive Surgery, Yale School of Medicine, 330 Cedar Street, Boardman Building 3rd Floor, New Haven, CT 06510, USA
* Corresponding author.
*E-mail address:* Furibe@uchc.edu

Oral Maxillofacial Surg Clin N Am 32 (2020) 297–307
https://doi.org/10.1016/j.coms.2020.01.011

which aim to reapproximate the maxillary alveolar segments in order to reduce tension on the repaired lip and improve nasal asymmetry. Though effective in the short term, their long-term effects on maxillary development and occlusion are debatable.[1-3]

## ORTHODONTICS AND ORTHOPEDIC CONSIDERATIONS IN BILATERAL AND UNILATERAL CLEFTS

Orthodontic needs of the patient with unilateral and bilateral cleft can vary depending on the extent of dentofacial deformities present. Common dental anomalies in cleft patients include microdontia, hypodontia, impacted dentition, supernumerary teeth, and transposition or ectopic dentition. Deficiency in the blood supply and mesenchymal support near the cleft site often result in congenitally missing maxillary lateral incisors.[4] Missing second premolars and supernumerary teeth distal to or within the cleft site are also commonly identified.[5,6] Increasing severity of the cleft has also been shown to result in more missing dentition in cases of both UCLP and BCLP.[6] Early detection is therefore necessary to prevent further disturbances in development.

Deficiency in the growth of the maxilla is also correlated with cleft severity and extent of postsurgical scarring.[7,8] As a result, restriction of the maxillary growth may be increased in BCLP patients. In UCLP, the maxillary lesser segment is significantly hypoplastic and displaced toward the side of the cleft (**Fig. 1**). Patients with UCLP also exhibit a constricted maxillary arch and anterior crossbite with or without a posterior crossbite on the cleft side. However, BCLP patients are more symmetric in nature, with increased collapse of both anterior and posterior maxillary segments and both anterior and posterior crossbites (**Fig. 2**).

### Orthodontic Intervention in the Early Mixed Dentition (7–8 Years Old)

Treatment goals during the early mixed dentition stage aim to improve the transverse and sagittal skeletal discrepancy through growth modification. The effectiveness of this intervention highly depends on the maturation status of the patient, with optimal results achieved before the patient reaches adolescence. During this time, orthopedic response is more favorable as the circummaxillary sutures are smooth with minimal interdigitation.[9] Although treatment can begin in the primary dentition, relapse of the discrepancy is likely to recur with growth. Therefore, early treatment is contraindicated because retreatment is often required.

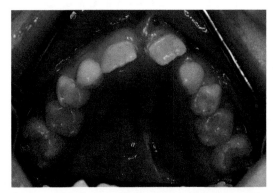

**Fig. 1.** Occlusal view of a patient with UCLP on the left side. Collapse of lesser maxillary segment toward the cleft is observed.

### Correction of transverse discrepancies

The collapsed posterior segments of the cleft lip and palate require transverse expansion to achieve an ideal arch form in preparation for alveolar bone grafting. Ideal expansion eliminates posterior crossbites by maximizing skeletal effects while minimizing any dental side effects.

In the early mixed dentition, both rapid and slow expanders can be used to correct for the transverse deficiency in the maxillary arch.[10] Although conventional expanders are often used to produce expansion in both the anterior and posterior regions of the arch, cleft patients often present with more severe constriction in the anterior maxilla. Therefore, modifications to the conventional rapid palatal expansion (RME) appliance (**Fig. 3**) have been made to allow for customized expansion in the anterior and posterior regions depending on the patient's needs.[11,12]

Expansion of the maxillary arch also improves access to the cleft site for alveolar grafting once the patient is in the late mixed dentition. However,

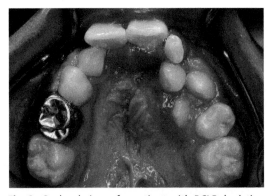

**Fig. 2.** Occlusal view of a patient with BCLP depicting a more symmetric but constricted arch anteriorly and posteriorly.

A

B

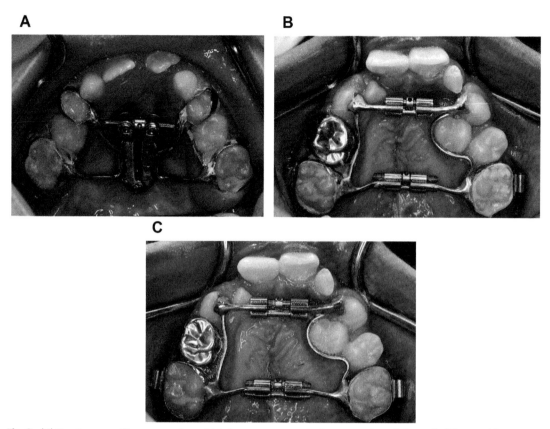

C

**Fig. 3.** (*A*) Fan-type maxillary expander, which favors a more anterior expansion of the arch. (*B*) RPE with 2 expansion screws to address differential expansion needs between the anterior and posterior regions of the arch. Passive appliance after insertion. (*C*) Active appliance with the anterior screw being activated more than the posterior one.

it is important that in patients with cleft lip and palate (CLP) there is little to no palatal suture remaining, which significantly reduces any resistance to expansion compared with that of non-cleft patients.[13] Care must be taken to minimize excessive expansion such that it exceeds the soft-tissue limitations and risks failure of future bone graft.[14] To prevent such a situation, slow expanders such as the quad helix type of appliance or W appliances may allow for a more controlled expansion and less tissue resistance.

### Correction of sagittal discrepancies

Mild to moderate midface deficiencies and anterior crossbites in the cleft patient can be treated with the use of the Delaire-type protraction facemask.[15,16] In addition to achieving maxillary protraction, the reciprocal force from the chin cup allows the downward and backward rotation of the mandible, minimizing the appearance of the retrusive maxilla. Furthermore, the location of the elastic pull from the facemask can be altered to achieve the desired movement. Given the vertical growth pattern tendency of CLP patients, efforts should aim to minimize any potential counterclockwise rotation of the maxilla. To counteract this, the direction of the elastics pull can be placed near the center of resistance of the maxilla (above the premolars), maximizing forward movement of the maxilla while minimizing opening of the bite.[17]

Because the maxillary arch of the cleft patient presents with sagittal and transverse deficiencies, maxillary expansion can be used in conjunction with facemask therapy. Studies have shown successful treatment of maxillary hypoplasia in UCLP patients with magnitude of advancement ranging from 0.8 mm to 4 mm.[15,16]

Another treatment protocol involving alternate rapid maxillary expansion and constriction (Alt-RAMEC) with facemask protraction has also been described in the literature.[18] Once the patient is in the late mixed dentition, this strategy may be used to achieve a greater degree of disarticulation of the circummaxillary sutures. Liou and Tsai[18] showed that alt-RAMEC allowed for maxillary displacement almost 3-times that of RME alone.

## Orthodontic Intervention in the Late Mixed Dentition (10–12 Years Old)

Treatment goals during the late mixed dentition stage aim to improve bone and periodontal support around the cleft site through alveolar bone grafting in preparation for future orthodontic tooth movement and/or prosthodontic rehabilitation. Once successful bone grafting is achieved, bone-anchored maxillary protraction may be performed during this stage to improve any remaining maxillary deficiency. Distraction of the hypoplastic maxilla may be used to correct severe skeletal discrepancies.

### Benefits of secondary alveolar bone grafting

Secondary alveolar bone grafting (ABG) is performed to stabilize the expanded maxillary segments and achieve a continuous alveolus in preparation for eruption of the permanent canine.[19] Successful grafting also augments bony support to allow for orthodontic tooth movement as well as prosthodontic rehabilitation of the cleft site. Closure of persistent oronasal and alveolar fistulas can also be achieved, minimizing leakage of food and fluids into the nasal passages. Secondary grafting further minimizes velopharyngeal dysfunction, resulting in improved speech formation and psychosocial development of the patient.[20]

### Timing of alveolar bone grafting

Proper timing of ABG is essential for optimal repair of the cleft site. Primary bone grafting (at the time of surgical lip repair) was commonly performed by cleft surgeons between the 1950s and 1970s. However, studies have since shown significant growth disturbances of the midface with such early grafting.[21] Secondary ABG is now advocated during the late mixed dentition to minimize interference with the maxillary growth.

The ideal time for secondary grafting is correlated with the development of the maxillary canine, when one-half to two-thirds of root formation has occurred and a thin layer of bone covers the crown.[22] Success rates of grafting after canine eruption are significantly diminished, with minimal improvement in crestal bone height and higher likelihood of graft resorption.[23,24] Continuous clinical and radiographic evaluations to monitor the patient's growth and development are therefore necessary throughout this period to ensure optimal timing of ABG.

Deciduous or supernumerary teeth that interfere with surgical access to the cleft site will need to be removed 2 to 3 months before grafting. Although extractions may be completed at the same time as ABG, studies have shown fewer complications in patients who had preoperative extractions.[25] Moreover, limited presurgical orthodontic treatment may be required to align severely malpositioned incisors before grafting to improve access to the cleft site and maximize grafting success.

Successful bone grafting is required before beginning orthodontic treatment. Limited cone-beam computed tomography (CBCT) imaging can confirm integrity of the bone graft. Tooth movement is recommended 3 months after successful grafting, but no later than 6 months, to allow for proper graft stimulation.[26] Delay in orthodontic treatment after grafting has been shown to result in relapse of the premaxilla and potential lingual collapse of the central incisor.[27]

### Orthopedics for midface deficiency in the late mixed dentition

**Bone-anchored maxillary protraction** Orthopedics in the late mixed dentition has been applied primarily through skeletal anchorage devices. There are 2 methods commonly used to protract the cleft maxilla: (1) miniplate-assisted facemask protraction and (2) bone-anchored protraction using intermaxillary elastics (BAMP). The former approach requires approximately 12 to 14 hours of wear with heavy forces induced by the elastics (500–1000 g). Effective protraction of the maxilla using a facemask with miniplate anchorage has been shown previously in both BCLP and UCLP, although less advancement is observed in patients with BCLP, likely as a result of increased postsurgical scar tissue.[28,29]

In cases of delayed orthopedic treatment or insufficient protraction of the hypoplastic maxilla with early treatment with tooth-anchored protraction facemask, BAMP can be initiated once the patient is in the late mixed dentition. With this method, the maxilla is moved forward using intraoral intermaxillary elastics attached to bone plates placed at the maxillary infrazygomatic crests and between the mandibular permanent canine and lateral incisors (**Fig. 4**). The elastics are applied continuously for 24 hours with low traction forces (100–250 g).

Successful maxillary protraction in the cleft patient has been shown using this approach.[30,31] Furthermore, the amount of forward displacement of the maxilla is comparable in cleft patients treated with bone-anchored maxillary protraction and those treated with miniplate-anchored facemask protraction.[30] Similar advancement has also been reported in cleft patients treated with BAMP therapy in comparison with non-cleft patients, suggesting that scar tissue and fibrosis do not interfere with protraction.[31]

A
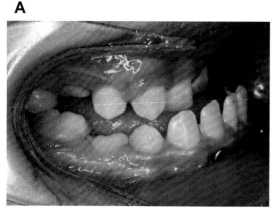

B
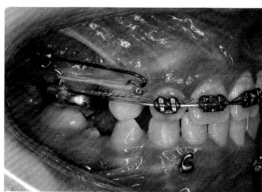

**Fig. 4.** An 11-year-old female patient with UCLP and significant underjet. (*A*) Sagittal view at the beginning of BAMP therapy with 24-h class III elastics. (*B*) One year of elastic wear from miniplates shows the significant maxillary protraction and normalization of the overjet.

Compared with conventional facemask therapy, BAMP minimizes dental side effects often seen with tooth-anchored protraction (ie, proclination of the upper incisors).[32] Furthermore, once anteroposterior (AP) correction of the hypoplastic maxilla is achieved the patient can immediately begin orthodontic treatment, resulting in decreased active treatment duration. In addition, this technique eliminates the need for patient compliance that is required in facemask protraction. Class III elastics can also be worn throughout fixed-appliance therapy and after AP correction to minimize potential relapse.

**Timing of bone-anchored maxillary protraction**
Ideal timing of BAMP depends on sufficient maxillary and mandibular bone thickness. Given the increased porosity of the maxillary bone, it is important to delay bone-anchored treatment until the late mixed dentition when there is sufficient increase in bone density to allow for mechanical retention of screws. This delayed approach also provides the patient and cleft team more time to address the remaining skeletal discrepancy.

*Orthopedics for midface deficiency in the late mixed dentition*
**Distraction osteogenesis** Distraction osteogenesis (DO) serves as an alternative treatment approach for the correction of severe maxillary deficiency in young patients with CLP. Compared with conventional Le Fort I advancement, DO can be initiated before the end of skeletal growth and is an attractive alternative for growing patients.[33]

Though effective, long-term stability of early DO in the cleft patient remains debatable. Because growth potential of the mandible is unpredictable, repeat distractions or orthognathic surgery may be

needed.[34] Overcorrection in growing children is also often recommended because of potential relapse (particularly in BCLP cases).

**Rehabilitative treatment of missing dentition**
Following successful bone grafting, esthetic rehabilitation of missing dentition in the cleft patient is required to help alleviate functional disturbances and improve the patient's quality of life. In cases of congenitally missing lateral incisors or other missing anterior dentition, treatment options often include space opening for prosthetic replacement (removable or fixed), orthodontic/surgical space closure for canine substitution, or autotransplantation of developing premolars. The treatment decision depends on the patient's existing skeletal pattern, dental relationship, size of cleft-dental gap, success of ABG, and personal preference.

**Canine substitution** Orthodontic gap closure and canine substitution is a common treatment choice for CLP patients with congenitally missing lateral incisors. With space closure, treatment can be started either concurrently with or immediately after bone grafting and does not require completion of growth as required with implant placement. Graft stimulation with orthodontic tooth movement also minimizes resorption of the grafted bone.[26,27] A healthier periodontium has been reported in cleft patients treated with canine substitution when compared with those with prosthetic lateral incisors.[35] Although extensive reshaping and restoration may be required, when done properly, canine substitution can provide esthetic results and greater patient satisfaction (**Fig. 5**).

When achieving space closure or narrowing of the residual cleft gap both orthodontic and surgical treatment modalities can be considered,

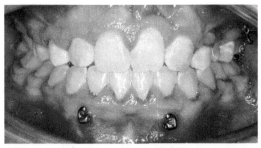

**Fig. 5.** A patient with UCLP on the left side with bilateral maxillary canine substitution for absent lateral incisors. Note the similar tooth morphology obtained from the canines in the replacement of the lateral incisors after contouring of the incisal, proximal and labial surfaces.

depending on the prosthodontic goals and extent of the gap. Advancement of the lesser segment can be effectively achieved through fixed-appliance therapy. However, cleft patients often present with large dental gaps as a result of presurgical expansion. In such cases, segmental osteotomies with concurrent bone grafting can be performed to close or narrow the gap (**Figs. 6** and **7**).[36]

Alveolar cleft closure by DO of the osteotomized segment posterior to the cleft site is an alternative option.[37] Tooth-borne and bone-borne DO devices have shown successful movement of the maxillary segment in BCLP and UCLP patients. Though effective, these options may be prohibitive for reasons of prolonged treatment time as well as potential soft-tissue irritation and patient discomfort from the distraction device. Moreover, significant

advancement of the posterior segment can be limited and may not address wide cleft gaps.

**Autotransplantation** Tooth autotransplantation serves as a predictable and effective option for the replacement of missing dentition (**Fig. 8**). Successful premolar transplantation to the bone graft area in patients with CLP has been reported in the literature.[38] With proper case selection and surgical technique, autotransplanted teeth can serve as a more natural restorative solution to achieving dental rehabilitation.

Benefits of autotransplantation include improved esthetic and functional results, preservation of the alveolar ridge, and increased patient satisfaction. Unlike implants, autotransplanted teeth maintain proprioceptive function and exhibit root development.[39] Therefore, autotransplanted teeth can benefit the growing patient and eliminate the need for future implant insertion once growth has ceased. Potentially lower treatment costs are also an added benefit in comparison with dental implants and other prosthetic restorations. Favorable long-term stability of autotransplanted teeth in cleft patients has also been described in the literature.[38,40]

### Orthodontic Intervention in the Permanent Dentition (18 Years Old and Upward)

Following growth cessation and eruption of the permanent dentition, a thorough evaluation of the patient's facial growth and development is required. Treatment during this phase aims to correct any residual maxillomandibular discrepancies (if present) and attain ideal dental alignment and occlusion. If

**A**                                        **B**

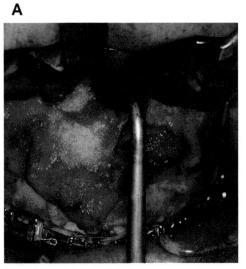
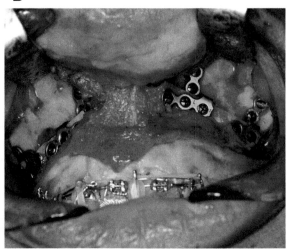

**Fig. 6.** (*A*, *B*) Segmental osteotomy procedure depicting the advancement of the posterior segment into the cleft with simultaneous bone grafting.

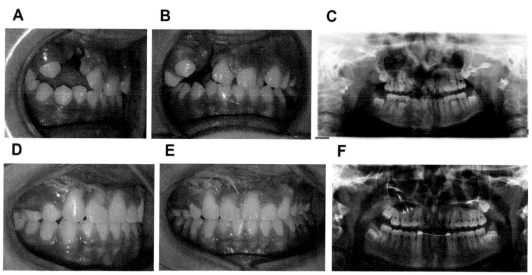

**Fig. 7.** Segmental osteotomy for patient with UCLP. (*A, B*) Presurgical intraoral photos. (*C*) Presurgical panoramic radiograph. (*D, E*) Post-treatment intraoral photos. (*F*) Panoramic radiograph after segmental osteotomy and orthodontics to close cleft. (*From* [*A*] Wilson AT, Wu RT, Sawh-Martinez R, et al. Segmental maxillary osteotomy to close wide alveolar clefts. J Oral Maxillofac Surg. 2019;77(4):850.e2; with permission; and [*C, E*] Wilson AT, Wu RT, Sawh-Martinez R, et al. Segmental maxillary osteotomy to close wide alveolar clefts. J Oral Maxillofac Surg. 2019;77(4):850.e3; with permission; and [*F*] Wilson AT, Wu RT, Sawh-Martinez R, et al. Segmental maxillary osteotomy to close wide alveolar clefts. J Oral Maxillofac Surg. 2019;77(4):850.e4; with permission.)

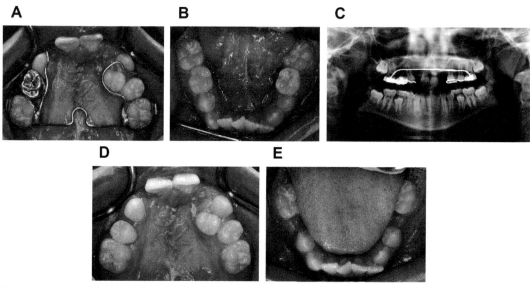

**Fig. 8.** A patient with BCLP with missing right second premolar and significant crowding in the mandible. The treatment plan included extraction of the second mandibular premolars and autotransplantation into the site of the missing right second premolar. The final orthodontic plan consisted of canine substitution of the missing maxillary lateral incisors. (*A*) Presurgical occlusal view of the maxilla. (*B*) Occlusal view of the crowded mandibular dentition before extraction of the second premolars. (*C*) Panoramic radiograph showing the missing maxillary lateral incisor and right second premolar. Mandibular second premolars are at the ideal time for autotransplantation, with approximately two-thirds of the roots formed; (*D*) Occlusal view of the autotransplanted mandibular right second premolar to the right maxillary second premolar site. (*E*) Occlusal view of the mandibular arch after extraction of the second premolars.

correction of midface retrusion was achieved through orthopedic traction in the early and mixed dentition, the patient may only need orthodontic treatment to correct for mild or moderate discrepancies. Replacement of any missing dentition may also be addressed during this stage with the rehabilitation options described previously. However, patients with severe skeletal deformities or those with relapse of the hypoplastic maxilla after early correction may require a combination of orthodontic treatment and orthognathic surgery.

### Preparation guidelines for orthognathic surgery

Effective presurgical planning by both the surgeon and orthodontist is essential in achieving successful surgical outcomes. Preoperative radiographic and clinical evaluation of the patient's skeletal and dental relationships is carried out by both the

surgeon and orthodontist. Extraoral photographs help determine deviations in the facial proportions and symmetry. Lateral cephalogram radiographs with tracings help assess the severity of maxillomandibular discrepancy in addition to dental and soft-tissue relationships. Finally, dental-cast analysis is used to determine the amount and type of maxillary and mandibular movements needed to achieve dentofacial harmony.

Although such two-dimensional methods for surgical planning are still used today, three-dimensional simulations using CBCT scans can serve as a more reliable and predictable tool to address the significant asymmetries and facial distortions often seen in UCLP and BCLP patients. Moreover, various studies have highlighted the benefits of virtual surgical planning in both the cleft and non-cleft patient, including increased surgical accuracy and reduced operation time.[41,42]

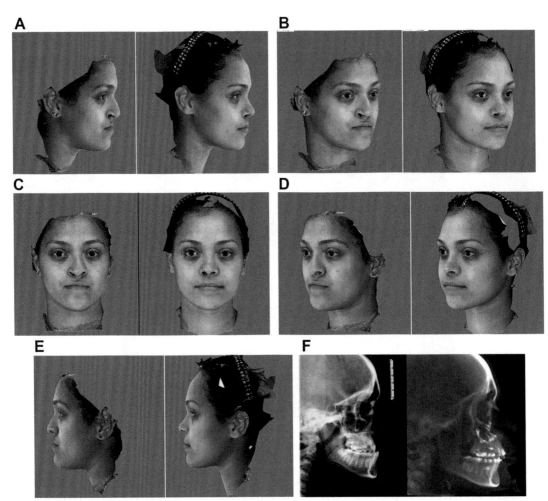

**Fig. 9.** Maxillary advancement with simultaneous segmental osteotomy to close UCLP with a surgery-first approach in an adolescent female patient. (*A–E*) Before and after extraoral photographs. (*F*) Pretreatment and postsurgical lateral cephalograms.

## Orthognathic surgery in the cleft patient

Orthognathic surgery in the cleft patient often requires presurgical orthodontics to achieve ideal alignment and eliminate major dental discrepancies. In limited cases, a surgery-first option may be elected. Cleft patients may also require maxillary advancement in addition to mandibular setback surgery depending on the severity of the skeletal discrepancy. Segmental Le Fort I osteotomies with advancement may be used to effectively correct the skeletal discrepancy, close a wide cleft-dental gap, and achieve fistula closure (**Fig. 9**). Concurrent with orthognathic surgery, lip revisions, and rhinoplasty may also be performed in some patients, although these procedures are often staged separately so as to minimize disturbance to the maxillary blood supply.

## Mandibular miniplates in orthognathic surgery

Patients may express some grade of maxillary relapse after surgical advancement. To mask this relapse and secure an adequate occlusal outcome, the orthodontist can place miniplates in the external oblique ridge of the mandible for lower arch distalization. This approach can be observed in **Fig. 10**. This patient had an edge-to-edge occlusion anteriorly that was not corrected by the prescribed class III elastics. Therefore, miniplates placed in the mandible served as an anchor to obtain a favorable occlusion.

A                    B

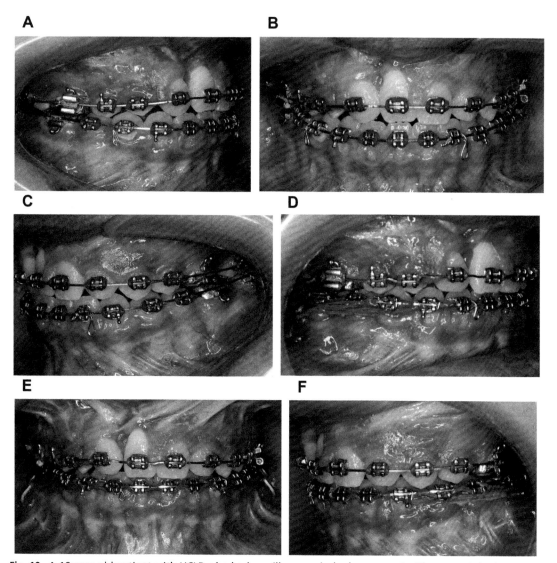

C                    D

E                    F

**Fig. 10.** A 16-year-old patient with UCLP who had maxillary surgical advancement with segmental osteotomy to close the right cleft. (*A–C*) Relapse observed 6 months after surgery, with the patient not complying with elastic wear. (*D–F*) Normal overjet achieved after 3 months of mandibular arch distalization with miniplates.

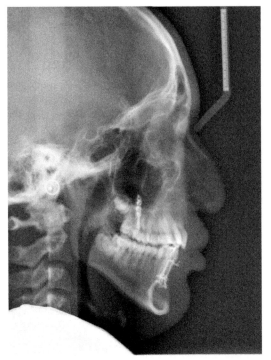

**Fig. 11.** Lateral cephalogram of a 13-year-old male patient after BAMP therapy. The patient wears class III elastics at nighttime from miniplates to maintain anteroposterior correction.

### Retention

The orthodontic retention protocol often involves traditional appliances such as Hawley retainers for the maxillary and mandibular arch. Alternatively, permanent lingual retention from canine to canine in the mandibular arch can also be used. To minimize skeletal relapse, patients previously treated with BAMP may retain their plate until full completion of growth for continuous orthopedic traction using class III elastics (**Fig. 11**) during the remnant growth period.

## SUMMARY

Orthodontic treatment of patients with UCLP and BCLP can be challenging. Treatment often requires both skeletal and dental correction of orofacial defects initiated at various stages of the patient's dental development. Early treatment methods focus on growth modification for correction of skeletal discrepancies, whereas later treatment is aimed toward dental rehabilitation of the cleft-dental gap. Successful management of the cleft patient ultimately requires extensive communication between the orthodontist and other members of the cleft team with the aim of achieving optimal dentofacial esthetics and meeting the patient's expectations.

## DISCLOSURE

The authors have nothing to disclose.

## REFERENCES

1. Clark SL, Teichgraeber JF, Fleshman RG, et al. Long-term treatment outcome of presurgical nasoalveolar molding in patients with unilateral cleft lip and palate. J Craniofac Surg 2011;22(1):333–6.
2. Shetty V, Agrawal RK, Sailer HF. Long-term effect of presurgical nasoalveolar molding on growth of maxillary arch in unilateral cleft lip and palate: randomized controlled trial. Int J Oral Maxillofac Surg 2017;46(8):977–87.
3. AlHayyan WA, Pani SC, Al Johar AJ, et al. The effects of presurgical nasoalveolar molding on the midface symmetry of children with unilateral cleft lip and palate: a long-term follow-up study. Plast Reconstr Surg Glob Open 2018;6(7):e1764.
4. Tsai TP, Huang CS, Huang CC, et al. Distribution patterns of primary and permanent dentition in children with unilateral complete cleft lip and palate. Cleft Palate Craniofac J 1998;35:154–60.
5. Shapira Y, Lubit E, Kuftinec MM. Congenitally missing second premolars in cleft lip and cleft palate children. Am J Orthod Dentofacial Orthop 1999;115(4):396–400.
6. Shapira Y, Lubit E, Kuftinec MM. Hypodontia in children with various types of clefts. Angle Orthod 2000;70(1):16–21.
7. Good PM, Mulliken JB, Padwa BL. Frequency of Le Fort I osteotomy after repaired cleft lip and palate or cleft palate. Cleft Palate Craniofac J 2007;44:396–401.
8. Normando AD, da Silva Filho OG, Capelozza Filho L. Influence of surgery on maxillary growth in cleft lip and/or palate patients. J Craniomaxillofac Surg 1992;20(3):111–8.
9. Melsen B, Melsen F. The postnatal development of the palatomaxillary region studied on human autopsy material. Am J Orthod 1982;82(4):329–42.
10. Vasant MR, Menon S, Kannan S. Maxillary expansion in cleft lip and palate using quad helix and rapid palatal expansion screw. Med J Armed Forces India 2009;65(2):150–3.
11. Figueiredo DS, Bartolomeo FU, Romualdo CR, et al. Dentoskeletal effects of 3 maxillary expanders in patients with clefts: a cone-beam computed tomography study. Am J Orthod Dentofacial Orthop 2014;146(1):73–81.
12. Garib D, Lauris RC, Calil LR, et al. Dentoskeletal outcomes of a rapid maxillary expander with differential opening in patients with bilateral cleft lip and palate: a prospective clinical trial. Am J Orthod Dentofacial Orthop 2016;150(4):564–74.
13. Pan X, Qian Y, Yu J, et al. Biomechanical effects of rapid palatal expansion on the craniofacial skeleton

with cleft palate: a three-dimensional finite element analysis. Cleft Palate Craniofac J 2007;44:149–54.

14. Shetye PR. Orthodontic management of patients with cleft lip and palate. APOS Trends Orthod 2016;6(28):1–6.

15. Buschang PH, Porter C, Genecov E, et al. Face mask therapy of preadolescents with unilateral cleft lip and palate. Angle Orthod 1994;64(2):145–50.

16. Dogan S. The effects of face mask therapy in cleft lip and palate patients. Ann Maxillofac Surg 2012;2(2):116–20.

17. Yepes E, Quintero P, Rueda ZM, et al. Optimal force for maxillary protraction facemask therapy in the early treatment of class III malocclusion. Eur J Orthod 2014;36(5):586–94.

18. Liou EJ, Tsai WC. A new protocol for maxillary protraction in cleft patients: repetitive weekly protocol of alternate rapid maxillary expansions and constrictions. Cleft Palate Craniofac J 2005;42(2):121–7.

19. Bergland O, Semb G, Abyholm FE. Elimination of the residual alveolar cleft by secondary bone grafting and subsequent orthodontic treatment. Cleft Palate J 1986;23:175–205.

20. Bureau S, Penko M, McFadden L. Speech outcome after closure of oronasal fistulas with bone grafts. J Oral Maxillofac Surg 2001;59(12):1408–13.

21. Friede H, Johanson B. A follow-up study of cleft children treated with primary bone grafting: orthodontic aspects. Scand J Plast Reconstr Surg 1974;8(1–2):88–103.

22. Lilja J. Alveolar bone grafting. Indian J Plast Surg 2009;42(Suppl):S110–5.

23. Calvo AM, Trindade-Suedam IK, da Silva Filho OG, et al. Increase in age is associated with worse outcomes in alveolar bone grafting in patients with bilateral complete cleft palate. J Craniofac Surg 2014;25(2):380–2.

24. Tuvey TA, Vig K, Moriarty J. Delayed bone grafting in the cleft maxilla and palate: a retrospective multidisciplinary analysis. Am J Orthod Dentofacial Orthop 1984;86(3):244–56.

25. Almasri M. Reconstruction of the alveolar cleft: effect of preoperative extraction of deciduous teeth at the sites of clefts on the incidence of postoperative complications. Br J Oral Maxillofac Surg 2012;50(2):154–6.

26. Yang C, Qian Y, Chen Z. Study on tooth movement after the alveolar bone grafting in patients with unilateral cleft lip and palate. J Craniofac Surg 2019;30(4):284–8.

27. Boyne PJ, Horford AS, Stringer DE. Prevention of relapse following cleft bone grafting and the future use of BMP cytokines to regenerate osseous clefts without grafting. In: Berkowitz S, editor. Cleft lip and palate: diagnosis and management. Berlin: Springer; 2006. p. 587–600.

28. On SW, Baek SH, Choi JY. Effect of long-term use of facemask with miniplate on maxillary protraction in patients with cleft lip and palate. J Craniofac Surg 2018;29(2):309–14.

29. Ahn HW, Kim KW, Yang IH, et al. Comparison of the effects of maxillary protraction using facemask and miniplate anchorage between unilateral and bilateral cleft lip and palate patients. Angle Orthod 2012;82:935–41.

30. Jahanbin A, Kazemian M, Eslami N, et al. Maxillary protraction with intermaxillary elastics to miniplates versus bone-anchored face-mask therapy in cleft lip and palate patients. J Craniofac Surg 2016;27(5):1247–52.

31. Yatabe M, Garib DG, Faco RAS. Bone-anchored maxillary protraction therapy in patients with unilateral complete cleft lip and palate: 3-dimensional assessment of maxillary effects. Am J Orthod Dentofacial Orthop 2017;152(3):327–35.

32. Ge YS, Liu J, Chen L, et al. Dentofacial effects of two facemask therapies for maxillary protraction. Angle Orthod 2012;82(6):1083–91.

33. Cheung LK, Chua HD. A meta-analysis of cleft maxillary osteotomy and distraction osteogenesis. Int J Oral Maxillofac Surg 2006;35(1):14–24.

34. Park YW, Kwon KJ, Kim MK. Long-term follow-up of early cleft maxillary distraction. Maxillofac Plast Reconstr Surg 2016;38(1):20.

35. Robertsson S, Mohlin B. The congenitally missing upper lateral incisor. A retrospective study of orthodontic space closure versus restorative treatment. Eur J Orthod 2000;22:697–710.

36. Wilson AT, Wu RT, Sawh-Martinez R, et al. Segmental maxillary osteotomy to close wide alveolar clefts. J Oral Maxillofac Surg 2019;77(4):850.e1–5.

37. Hegab AF. Closure of the alveolar cleft by bone segment transport using an intraoral tooth-borne custom-made distraction device. J Oral Maxillofac Surg 2012;70:337.

38. Aizenbud D, Zaks M, Abu-El-Naaj I, et al. Mandibular premolar autotransplantation in cleft affected patients: the replacement of congenital missing teeth as part of the cleft patient's treatment protocol. J Craniomaxillofac Surg 2013;41(5):371–81.

39. Paulsen HU, Andreasen JO. Eruption of premolars subsequent to autotransplantation. A longitudinal radiographic study. Eur J Orthod 1998;20(1):45–55.

40. Tanimoto K, Yanagida T, Tanne K. Orthodontic treatment with tooth transplantation for patients with cleft lip and palate. Cleft Palate Craniofac J 2010;47(5):499–506.

41. Lonic D, Pai BCJ, Yamaguchi K, et al. Computer-assisted orthognathic surgery for patients with cleft lip/palate: from traditional planning to three-dimensional surgical simulation. PLoS One 2016;11(3):e0152014.

42. Chin SJ, Wilde F, Neuhaus M. Accuracy of virtual surgical planning of orthognathic surgery with aid of CAD/CAM fabricated surgical splint-A novel 3D analyzing algorithm. J Craniomaxillofac Surg 2017;45(12):1962–70.

# Surgical-Orthodontic Considerations in Subcranial and Frontofacial Distraction

Richard A. Hopper, MD, MS[a], Hitesh Kapadia, DDS, PhD[b],
Srinivas M. Susarla, DMD, MD, MPH[c],*

## KEYWORDS

- Le Fort III osteotomy • Le Fort II osteotomy • Monobloc osteotomy • Subcranial distraction
- Counterclockwise craniofacial distraction • Frontofacial advancement
- Syndromic craniosynostosis

## KEY POINTS

- Distraction osteogenesis can be safely used for subcranial (Le Fort II, Le Fort III) or frontofacial (monobloc) advancements; proper orthodontic-surgical coordination is critical for a successful result.
- Midface distraction at the Le Fort III level is a valuable tool for managing the midface deficiency when the degree of hypoplasia is uniform across the midface (eg, Crouzon syndrome).
- Midface distraction osteogenesis at the Le Fort II level is useful for management of nasomaxillary hypoplasia (eg, Binder syndrome) or, when done in conjunction with zygomatic repositioning, for management of differential hypoplasia of the central midface relative to the orbitozygomatic complex (eg, Apert syndrome, achondroplasia).
- Frontofacial distraction can be used for management of midface hypoplasia in the context of anterior cranial vault constriction (eg, syndromic midface hypoplasia in the setting of intracranial hypertension). Monobloc frontofacial distraction advances the frontal bone and midface as a single unit.
- Synchronous counterclockwise rotation of the maxillomandibular complex is an emerging technique for management of complex hypoplasia involving the midface and mandible (eg, Treacher Collins syndrome).

## BACKGROUND

Distraction osteogenesis, initially pioneered for management of limb-length discrepancies, has been a major innovation in craniomaxillofacial surgery.[1–5] Although craniofacial distraction was initially described for management of mandibular hypoplasia, the technique has been effectively applied to myriad craniofacial differences, including midface deficiency, craniosynostosis, dentoalveolar hypoplasia, and management of hypertelorism. The shortcomings and morbidity of conventional osteotomies for management of complex subcranial and frontofacial deformities

Ethics Statement: All guidelines in the Declaration of Helsinki were followed in the course of this work. Consent was obtained for the use of clinical photographs.

[a] Craniofacial Center, Division of Plastic and Craniofacial Surgery, Seattle Children's Hospital, 4800 Sand Point Way NE, Seattle, WA 98105, USA; [b] Craniofacial Center, Division of Craniofacial Orthodontics, Seattle Children's Hospital, 4800 Sand Point Way NE, Seattle, WA 98105, USA; [c] Craniofacial Center, Divisions of Craniofacial and Plastic Surgery and Oral-Maxillofacial Surgery, Seattle Children's Hospital, 4800 Sand Point Way NE, Seattle, WA 98105, USA
* Corresponding author.
*E-mail address:* SRINIVAS.SUSARLA@SEATTLECHILDRENS.ORG

Oral Maxillofacial Surg Clin N Am 32 (2020) 309–320
https://doi.org/10.1016/j.coms.2020.01.005
1042-3699/20/© 2020 Elsevier Inc. All rights reserved.

have been long recognized: length of operations, blood loss, hospital stay, necessity for bone grafting, inadequate soft tissue results, infection, and relapse.[1–5] There is an increasing volume of data demonstrating the immediate efficacy and stability of subcranial and frontofacial distraction for management of complex morphologic deficiencies affecting the upper two-thirds of the face.[6–14] Although perioperative morbidity rates for subcranial and frontofacial distraction remain significant due to the complexity of the regional anatomy and procedural details, in many centers, distraction procedures have replaced conventional osteotomies for management of upper and midface deficiency.[7–17]

## GOALS OF SUBCRANIAL AND FRONTOFACIAL DISTRACTION

The primary goal of subcranial or frontofacial distraction osteogenesis is to reposition the hypoplastic upper or midfacial skeleton to correct (or overcorrect) the developmental deficiency. Recognition of the specific deficiencies by anatomic region (anterior cranial vault, orbitozygomatic complex, nasal pyramid, and maxilla) is critical for treatment success. Osteotomy patterns are tailored to the morphologic characteristics that need to be addressed (**Fig. 1**).

In a patient with Crouzon syndrome, there is a proportionate midface discrepancy—the degree of hypoplasia in the orbitozygomatic region matches that of the nasomaxillary complex; the Crouzon phenotype is a morphologically normal midface in an abnormal position (**Fig. 2**). Correction at this level, via a Le Fort III distraction, is primarily related to improving the relationship between the infraorbital rim and anterior cornea (correcting exorbitism).

In contrast, the patient with Apert syndrome will have a midface deficiency that is disproportionate—the central midface hypoplasia is more profound than the zygomatic hypoplasia. The Apert phenotype is a morphologically abnormal midface in an abnormal position (**Fig. 3**). Correction in this context is differential between the lateral and central midface. Correction of exorbitism is accomplished with zygomatic repositioning; the central vertical and sagittal midface deficiency is addressed with Le Fort II distraction.

Patients with syndromic midface hypoplasia with concomitant intracranial hypertension related to cranial vault constriction present a more challenging clinical picture. Morphologic characteristics include frontal retrusion, exorbitism, and concomitant midface hypoplasia (**Fig. 4**). In this context, frontofacial advancement via monobloc distraction is an effective approach for addressing the anterior cranial vault and midface deficiencies simultaneously.

Complex clockwise rotational deformities involving the mid- and lower-facial skeleton are characterized by bimaxillary retrognathism with a class II skeletal pattern, long anterior face height, steep mandibular and palatal planes, and airway obstruction. For this phenotype, synchronous counterclockwise rotation of the maxillomandibular complex is an effective technique for correcting the maxillomandibular position, palatal and mandibular planes, anterior and posterior face heights, and improving airway dynamics (**Fig. 5**).

## TREATMENT PLANNING

As with any surgical procedure, appropriate preoperative evaluation, diagnosis, and treatment planning based on sound principles are the keys to a successful result.[18] A comprehensive dentofacial assessment, including both the hard and soft tissues, is paramount. Objective assessment of cranial morphology, globe position, malar projection, nasal morphology, maxillary and mandibular sagittal and vertical positioning, as well as a

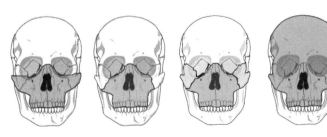

**Fig. 1.** Different patterns of osteotomy designs for correction of midface hypoplasia. The Le Fort III osteotomy (*left*) will result in separation of the entire midface from the cranial base, allowing advancement of the orbitozygomatic and nasomaxillary complexes as a single unit. The Le Fort II osteotomy (*middle left*) will allow for advancement of the nasomaxillary complex and may be combined with bilateral inverted-L mandibular osteotomies for synchronous counterclockwise craniofacial rotation. Segmentation of the Le Fort III osteotomy (Le Fort II with zygomatic repositioning) can allow for differential movement of the orbitozygomatic complex relative to the nasomaxillary segment (*middle right*). Severe midface deficiency in the setting of cranial vault constriction can be addressed with simultaneous fronto-orbital and Le Fort III advancement (monobloc advancement, right).

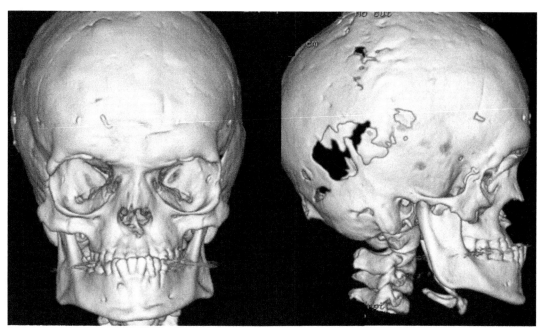

**Fig. 2.** Midface hypoplasia Crouzon syndrome. The midface deficiency is evenly distributed between the central and lateral midface. Clinically, this will be evident with poor malar support, exorbitism, and a class III profile. Correction of this specific midface morphology can be reliably accomplished with Le Fort III level distraction.

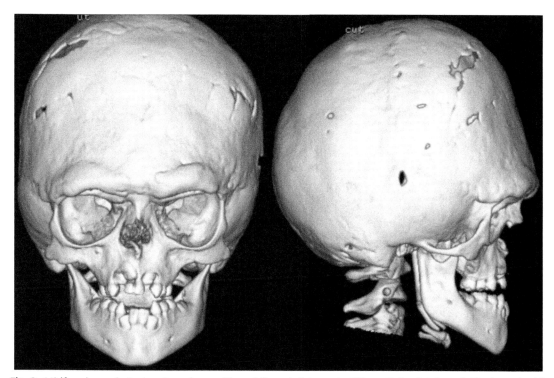

**Fig. 3.** Midface hypoplasia Apert syndrome. The midface deficiency is differentially distributed. The lateral orbi-tozyomgatic regions are hypoplastic, which is clinically evident as poor malar support and exorbitism. The central midface exhibits vertical and sagittal hypoplasia that is more severe than the lateral midface hypoplasia. Differential correction is indicated with zygomatic repositioning and Le Fort II level distraction with a downward and forward vector.

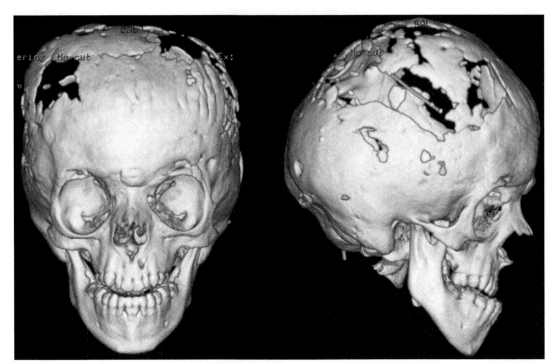

**Fig. 4.** Frontofacial dysmorphology in a patient with Crouzon syndrome who presented with multiple cranial defects, obstructive sleep apnea (AHI 62.6), intracranial hypertension, frontal and supraorbital retrusion, malignant proptosis, and midface hypoplasia. Management of the midface deformity in the context of anterior cranial vault constriction can be accomplished with monobloc frontofacial distraction.

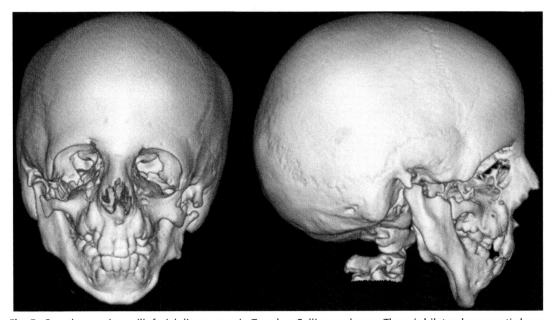

**Fig. 5.** Complex craniomaxillofacial discrepancy in Treacher Collins syndrome. There is bilateral zygomatic hypoplasia, bimaxillary retrognathism, a long anterior face height, and steep palatal and mandibular plane angles. This constellation of skeletal differences is associated with clockwise rotation of the mid- and lower-face and is amenable to correction with counterclockwise craniofacial distraction (C3DO) using a Le Fort II osteotomy with concomitant bilateral mandibular osteotomies and subsequent synchronous maxillomandibular distraction.

detailed intraoral assessment, focusing on hygiene, presence/absence of teeth, state of the dentition, crowding, transverse relationships, and occlusal plane orientation is necessary. Ophthalmologic assessment is an important adjunct in patients with exorbitism and those at risk for intracranial hypertension. Neurosurgical assessment is critical for patients undergoing frontofacial procedures.

Three-dimensional computed tomographic scans are critical for both diagnosis and treatment. Three-dimensional visualization of the specific anatomy is necessary to identify the specific morphologic deficiencies, plan appropriate distraction vectors, safely execute osteotomies and device placement, and overcome anatomic challenges such as persistent bony defects, shunts, sensory nerves, and developing dentition. Dental models (cast or digital) complement imaging modalities in this regard and remain essential for evaluating potential occlusal interferences

and for splint fabrication. Virtual surgical planning is used in many cases and affords an opportunity to visualize, in all three dimensions, the proposed skeletal movements and their impact on cephalometric parameters (**Fig. 6**).

The goals of treatment should be clearly established early in planning, with a focus on treatment plans tailored to the specific characteristics of the midface deficiency. Patients undergoing distraction procedures at the Le Fort II or Le Fort III levels are frequently in the mixed dentition. In this population, maxillary expansion and leveling of the occlusal plane may be required before surgical intervention. Pediatric dental assessment is necessary to manage active decay and reinforce the importance of excellent oral hygiene.

Patients undergoing frontofacial distraction procedures are frequently medically complex and require a collaborative, team-centered approach, including a craniofacial surgeon, neurosurgeon, ophthalmologist, orthodontist, and pediatric

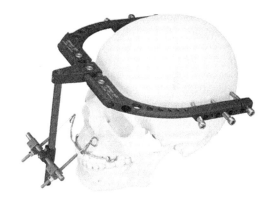

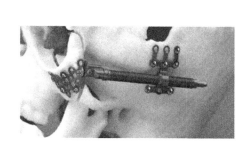

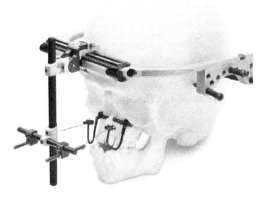

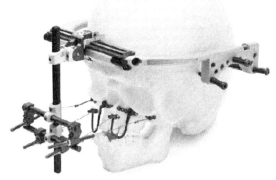

**Fig. 6.** Midface distraction appliances can be internal (*top left*)[24] or external. External distraction devices for midface distraction can be tooth-borne (*top right*)[25] or bone-borne (*bottom left*).[26] Additional fixation posts, typically placed in the lateral orbitozygomatic region (*bottom right*) help control the upper midface and prevent rotation of the distracted segment.[25] Tooth-borne devices require a prefabricated splint.

dentist. Although there remains controversy regarding early monobloc procedures (<2 years of age), older patients undergoing frontofacial advancements have dental needs similar to patients in the mixed dentition undergoing subcranial midface advancements. Preoperative planning for frontofacial distraction should take into account the specific cranial dysmorphology, including the presence of cranial defects and shunts. Coordinated treatment planning frequently allows for custom alloplastic cranioplasty to address cranial defects at the time of frontofacial osteotomies.

## DISTRACTION DEVICES

The distraction apparatus (**Fig. 7**) can be internal (directly affixed to bone) or external (halo device). Internal devices can be used to span the osteotomy gap without a splint, with fixation placed above and below the osteotomy or with a splint, with the inferior plate limb affixed to the splint. Similarly, external devices can be subdivided into those that use tooth-borne splints versus bone-borne fixation to connect to the external framework. Practitioner preferences vary in the choice of device, and each type has specific advantages and disadvantages. Purported advantages of external devices are related to the relative ease of placement, with less extensive subperiosteal dissection necessary, as well as differential forces (can "push" and "pull"), and, perhaps most importantly, 3-dimensional control of movement vectors. These advantages must

be weighed against the patient's tolerance for a cumbersome device that may become loose or dislodged and the risks of pin site infections. Internal devices are generally well hidden and placed closer to the primary osteotomy sites, theoretically reducing torque. However, placement is more challenging and requires extensive periosteal stripping, more significant staged procedures for device placement and removal, and distraction may be limited both in terms of magnitude and direction.

## SPLINT FABRICATION AND APPLICATION

With tooth-borne external midface distraction, a prefabricated occlusal splint is necessary (**Fig. 8**).[13,19,20] The splint is fabricated by using an orthodontic headgear bow as a framework within an acrylic occlusal registration. The internal wire is used to conform to the dentoalveolar morphology of the maxilla; the external wire is bent at 90-degree angle to accommodate outrigger hooks. The height of the outrigger hooks depends on both the patient's age and the planned distraction vector. The transverse dimension between the external wire limbs is slightly wider than the alar base width. The sagittal position of the external framework relative to the acrylic plate is based on the patient's lip thickness. The internal wire is embedded within a self-curing dental acrylic resin. The completed splint is then polished, both for patient comfort and to remove surface irregularities that are prone to plaque

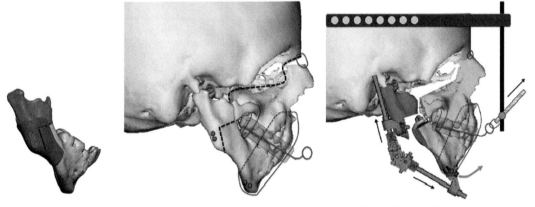

**Fig. 7.** Virtual surgical planning is an important adjunct for management of complex maxillomandibular deformities. Precise 3-dimensional visualization of the pertinent anatomy allows the surgeon to plan osteotomies and, when needed, fabricate cutting guides (left: cutting template for inverted-L osteotomies for counterclockwise craniofacial distraction osteogenesis (C3DO), with guide holes for transpharyngeal pin placement). Projected movements along the planned vector can be demonstrated, with associated measurement of cephalometric changes (middle and right: virtual surgical plan depicting pre- and post-distraction positions for C3DO). (*From* Hopper RA, Kapadia H, Susarla S, et al. Counterclockwise craniofacial distraction osteogenesis for tracheostomy-dependent children with Treacher Collins syndrome. Plast Reconstr Surg. 2018;142(2):447–57; with permission.)

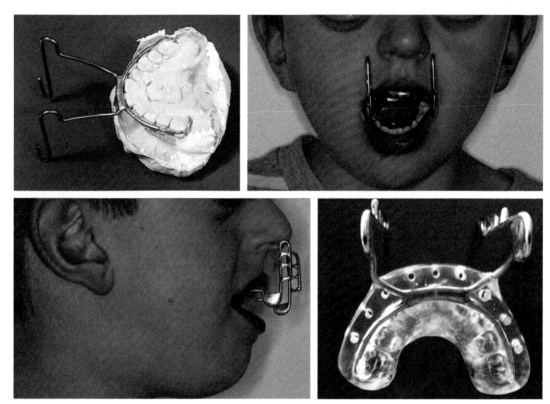

**Fig. 8.** Splint fabrication for external midface distraction. An orthodontic headgear bow is used for the framework. The internal wire is adapted to the maxillary arch form; the external wire is bent at a 90-degree angle to accommodate the outrigger hooks (*top left*). Proper orientation of the external framework requires meticulous attention. The width between the vertical limbs should be slightly larger than the alar base width (*top right*). The sagittal position of the bend should account for the upper lip thickness (*bottom left*). The final acrylated splint (*bottom right*).

accumulation. Intraoperatively, the splint is cemented to the maxillary dentition using a light-cured glass ionomer cement. In patients with oligodontia or where additional stability is otherwise needed, circum-zygomatic and circum-piriform wires (26-gauge) can be used to reinforce the splint and prevent dislodgement during activation. Once the splint is affixed to the teeth, it is connected to the rigid external device frame via 26-gauge stainless steel wires to the transverse bar. The vertical rod attachment can then be adjusted to achieve the appropriate height for the planned distraction vector.[13]

With Le Fort II and Le Fort III distraction procedures, the center of resistance for midface advancement is located slightly above the midpoint between the maxillary occlusal plane and nasion.[19,20] Application of the distraction force at this level will reliably advance the upper midface without affecting the occlusal plane. Pull of the pterygomasseteric sling tends to inferiorly reposition the posterior aspect of the Le Fort II or Le Fort III segment—if this is not accounted for,

an anterior open bite will result from counterclockwise rotation of the midface (ie, if the distraction force is too low). Conversely, a distraction force applied too high will result in clockwise rotation of the midface complex, resulting in overadvancement of the orbitozygomatic regions and possible enophthalmos.

For frontofacial advancements, the center of rotation will be located higher in the midface, resulting in a longer lever arm between the occlusal plane and center of rotation. Rotational movements are less frequently problematic in this group, due to the presence of additional stabilization posts within the lateral midface, but the vector of distraction needs to be continually assessed with serial lateral cephalograms, to ensure a vector parallel to the Frankfort horizontal.

In patients undergoing synchronous counterclockwise craniofacial distraction procedures, a Le Fort II osteotomy is performed in conjunction with bilateral mandibular inverted-L osteotomies.[14] A custom acrylic occlusal splint, similar to that used for external midface distraction, but adapted to include the mandibular dentition, is affixed to the teeth, and the patient is placed into maxillomandibular fixation with transpalatal and circummandibular wires (26-gauge). The splint construct is then wired to the activation arms with a 45-degree upward vector relative to the Frankfort horizontal.

## PERIOPERATIVE ORTHODONTIC TREATMENT

*During distraction*: once the planned osteotomies are completed and the prefabricated occlusal splint is affixed to the midface, the patient will have a latency period of approximately 5 days. The device is then activated at a rate of 0.5 mm twice a day. Distraction is complete when the predetermined endpoints have been achieved. With Le Fort III distraction, this is predicated on the lateral orbitozygomatic contour and correction of exorbitism (**Fig. 9**). With Le Fort II distraction, this is based on the nasal length and vertical height of the central midface (**Fig. 10**).[13] For frontofacial advancement, the distraction endpoints are determined by the position of the external orbit relative to the anterior cornea, frontal bone projection, and maxillary incisor position (**Fig. 11**). In growing patients, a goal overjet of 5 to 6 mm following subcranial or frontofacial advancement may also be considered as a treatment goal. With counterclockwise craniofacial rotation, active distraction is continued until the palatal plane is normalized (sella-nasion to palatal plane angle of 7°, **Fig. 12**).[14]

Following distraction progress with serial lateral cephalograms is critical during the active phase, as incorrect or inadequate vectors and problems with splint adaptation can be addressed. As discussed earlier, incorrect vertical positioning of the distraction force in the Le Fort II or III segment can result in undesirable counterclockwise or clockwise occlusal plane rotations. Placement of temporary anchorage devices in the midline mandible and elastic traction during activation can be helpful to address these specific vector issues. Orthodontic bone anchors are similarly useful adjuncts for vector control in Le Fort II distraction procedures as well as counterclockwise maxillomandibular rotations.

## POSTDISTRACTION ORTHODONTIC TREATMENT

Following completion of active distraction, patients will enter a consolidation phase (average 8 weeks). Once formation of bony generate is confirmed radiographically (most evident at the pterygomaxillary junction), the devices are removed. Postsurgical orthodontic treatment is

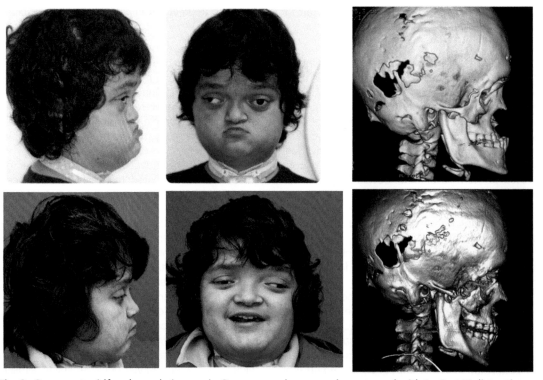

**Fig. 9.** Congruent midface hypoplasia seen in Crouzon syndrome can be managed with Le Fort III distraction.

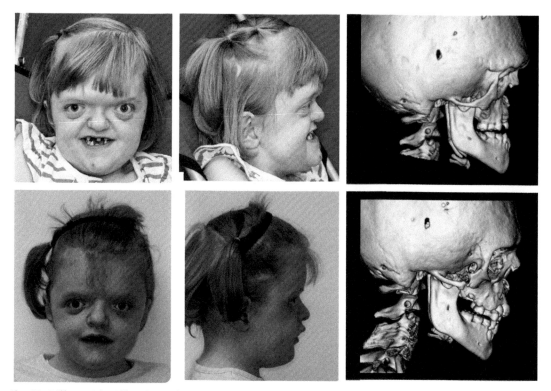

**Fig. 10.** Differential midface hypoplasia seen in Apert syndrome is appropriately addressed with Le Fort II distraction and zygomatic repositioning.

then undertaken. In many instances, postsurgical orthodontic care for the patient following midface distraction is similar to nonsurgical orthodontic care.

For patients undergoing midface distraction procedures in the mixed dentition, it is paramount to monitor growth of the midface relative to the mandible, as well as to follow dental eruption. There is evidence that subcranial midface osteotomies in younger patients results in disruptions in maxillary molar development and eruption.[10] Families should be counseled regarding this possibility preoperatively, and molar development should be carefully monitored in mixed dentition patients

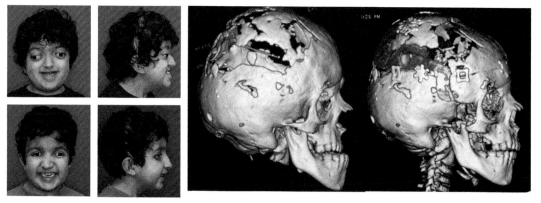

**Fig. 11.** This patient with Crouzon syndrome presented with large calvarial defects, intracranial hypertension, malignant proptosis, supraorbital retrusion, midface hypoplasia, and obstructive sleep apnea (AHI 67). The anterior cranial vault constriction and midface hypoplasia were addressed simultaneously with a monobloc frontofacial distraction. Postoperatively, the facial proportions were improved, with adequate globe protection. Postoperative polysomnography demonstrated substantial improvement in sleep-disordered breathing (AHI 3.7).

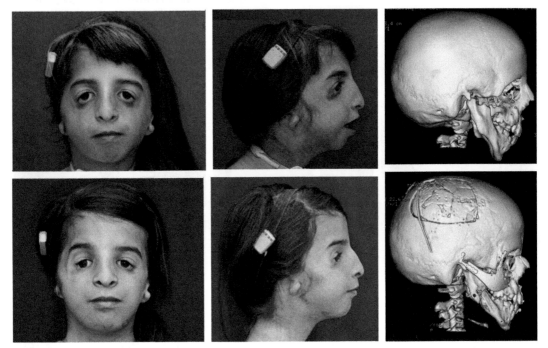

**Fig. 12.** The clockwise rotation deformity seen in Treacher Collins syndrome is managed with synchronous coun-terclockwise rotation distraction of the maxillomandibular complex, accomplished via Le Fort II and bilateral inverted-L mandibular osteotomies. In this patient, construction of the zygomas with autologous cranial bone graft was completed at the time of device removal. (*From* Hopper RA, Kapadia H, Susarla S, et al. Counterclock-wise craniofacial distraction osteogenesis for tracheostomy-dependent children with Treacher Collins syndrome. Plast Reconstr Surg. 2018;142(2):447–57; with permission.)

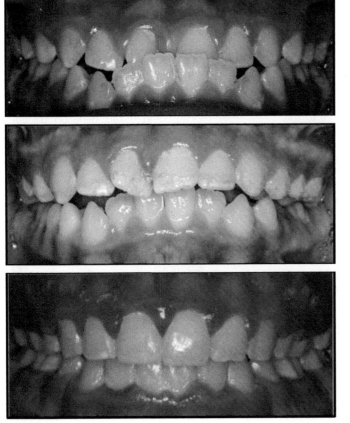

**Fig. 13.** Preoperative occlusion in a pa-tient with achondroplasia (*top*). Post-distraction occlusion following Le Fort II osteotomy with zygomatic reposi-tioning (*middle*); the midface position is overcorrected relative to the mandible, with positive overjet at the incisors. At skeletal maturity, the pa-tient underwent Le Fort I and bilateral mandibular sagittal split osteotomies for correction of the residual dentoske-letal discrepancy (*bottom*). (*From* Hop-per RA, Kapadia H, Susarla SM. Le Fort II Distraction With Zygomatic Repositioning: A Technique for Differential Correction of Midface Hypoplasia. J Oral Maxillofac Surg. 2018 Sep;76(9):2002.e1–14; with permission.)

undergoing subcranial distraction procedures. The available evidence demonstrates that although the distracted midface does not significantly relapse, growth is unpredictable and many patients undergoing subcranial midface advancement in the mixed dentition may require definitive orthognathic surgery at skeletal maturity. In this context, the goals of subcranial advancement established preoperatively are paramount. Anticipation of the need for occlusal and lower midface correction at skeletal maturity is necessary for appropriate treatment planning and patient/family counseling (**Fig. 13**).[5,21–23]

## SUMMARY

When properly planned and executed, subcranial advancement at the Le Fort II-III levels (including segmental movements and synchronous maxillomandibular counterclockwise rotations) and frontofacial distraction can be used to correct a wide array of craniomaxillofacial deformities. Focused attention on the specific morphologic characteristics of the patient, as well as an assessment of growth, and specific goals for distraction endpoints are necessary to ensure an optimal outcome.

## DISCLOSURE

Dr R.A. Hopper shares patent royalties with KLS Martin. The other authors have nothing to disclose.

## REFERENCES

1. McCarthy JG, Stelnicki EJ, Mehrara BJ, et al. Distraction osteogenesis of the craniofacial skeleton. PlastReconstr Surg 2001;107(7):1812–27.
2. Winters R, Tatum SA. Craniofacial distraction osteogenesis. Facial Plast Surg Clin North Am 2014;22(4):653–64.
3. Hopper RA. New trends in cranio-orbital and midface distraction for craniofacial dysostosis. Curr Opin Otolaryngol Head Neck Surg 2012;20(4):298–303.
4. Forrest CR, Hopper RA. Craniofacial syndromes and surgery. Plast Reconstr Surg 2013;131(1):86e–109e.
5. Taylor JA, Bartlett SP. What's new in syndromiccraniosynostosis surgery? Plast Reconstr Surg 2017;140(1):82e–93e.
6. Britto JA, Greig A, Abela C, et al. Frontofacial surgery in children and adolescents: techniques, indications, outcomes. Semin Plast Surg 2014;28(3):121–9.
7. Swennen G, Schliephake H, Dempf R, et al. Craniofacial distraction osteogenesis: a review of the literature: Part 1: clinical studies. Int J Oral Maxillofac Surg 2001;30(2):89–103.
8. Gwanmesia I, Jeelani O, Hayward R, et al. Frontofacial advancement by distraction osteogenesis: a long-term review. Plast Reconstr Surg 2015;135(2):553–60.
9. Glass GE, Ruff CF, Crombag GAJC, et al. The role of bipartition distraction in the treatment of apert syndrome. Plast Reconstr Surg 2018;141(3):747–50.
10. Way BLM, Khonsari RH, Karunakaran T, et al. Correcting exorbitism by monoblocfrontofacial advancement in crouzon-pfeiffer syndrome: an age-specific, time-related, controlled study. Plast Reconstr Surg 2019;143(1):121e–32e.
11. Hopper RA, Prucz RB, Iamphongsai S. Achieving differential facial changes with Le Fort III distraction osteogenesis: the use of nasal passenger grafts, cerclage hinges, and segmental movements. Plast Reconstr Surg 2012;130(6):1281–8.
12. Hopper RA, Kapadia H, Morton T. Normalizing facial ratios in apert syndrome patients with Le Fort II midface distraction and simultaneous zygomatic repositioning. Plast Reconstr Surg 2013;132(1):129–40.
13. Hopper RA, Kapadia H, Susarla S, et al. Counterclockwise craniofacial distraction osteogenesis for tracheostomy-dependent children with treachercollins syndrome. Plast Reconstr Surg 2018;142(2):447–57.
14. Hopper RA, Kapadia H, Susarla SM. Le Fort II distraction with zygomatic repositioning: a technique for differential correction of midface hypoplasia. J Oral Maxillofac Surg 2018;76(9):2002.e1-14.
15. Zhang RS, Lin LO, Hoppe IC, et al. Retrospective review of the complication profile associated with 71 subcranial and transcranialmidface distraction procedures at a single institution. Plast Reconstr Surg 2019;143(2):521–30.
16. Shetye PR, Davidson EH, Sorkin M, et al. Evaluation of three surgical techniques for advancement of the midface in growing children with syndromiccraniosynostosis. Plast Reconstr Surg 2010;126(3):982–94.
17. Patel PA, Shetye PR, Warren SM, et al. Five-year follow-up of midface distraction in growing children with syndromiccraniosynostosis. Plast Reconstr Surg 2017;140(6):794e–803e.
18. Wirthlin JO, Shetye PR. Orthodontist's role in orthognathic surgery. Semin Plast Surg 2013;27(3):137–44.
19. Shetye PR, Grayson BH, McCarthy JG. Le Fort III distraction: controlling position and path of the osteotomizedmidface segment on a rigid platform. J Craniofac Surg 2010;21(4):1118–21.
20. Shetye PR, Giannoutsos E, Grayson BH, et al. Le Fort III distraction: Part I. Controlling position and vectors of the midface segment. Plast Reconstr Surg 2009;124(3):871–8.
21. Caterson EJ, Shetye PR, Grayson BH, et al. Surgical management of patients with a history of early Le Fort III advancement after they have attained

skeletal maturity. Plast Reconstr Surg 2013;132(4): 592e–601e.

22. Susarla SM, Mundinger GS, Kapadia H, et al. Subcranial and orthognathic surgery for obstructive sleep apnea in achondroplasia. J Craniomaxillofac Surg 2017;45(12):2028–34.

23. Bastidas N, Mackay DD, Taylor JA, et al. Analysis of the long-term outcomes of nonsyndromicbicoronalsynostosis. PlastReconstr Surg 2012;130(4):877–83.

24. Image adapted from: Internal midface distractor. DepuySynthes Inc. Available at: http://synthes.vo.llnwd.net/o16/LLNWMB8/INT%20Mobile/Synthes%20International/Product%20Support%20Material/legacy_Synthes_PDF/DSEM-CMF-0516-0131_LR.pdf. Accessed December 10, 2019.

25. Image adapted from: External Midfacedistraction system. DepuySynthes Inc. Available at: http://synthes.vo.llnwd.net/o16/LLNWMB8/US%20Mobile/Synthes%20North%20America/Product%20Support%20Materials/Technique%20Guides/DSUSCMF10160637_ExMidDisSys_TG_150dpi.pdf. Accessed December 10, 2019.

26. Image adapted from: RED II distraction system. KLS Martin Inc. Available at: http://www.klsmartinnorthamerica.com/products/distraction-devices/lefort-iii-and-monobloc/red-ii-distraction-system/. Accessed December 10, 2019.

# Selected Orthodontic Principles for Management of Cranio-Maxillofacial Deformities

Timothy J. Tremont, DMD, MS[a],*, Jeffrey C. Posnick, DMD, MD[b,c,d]

## KEYWORDS

- Cranio-maxillofacial abnormalities • Cleft lip and palate • WALA ridge • Smiling profile
- Glabella vertical • Maxillary transverse • Curve of Spee

## KEY POINTS

- The WALA ridge is a useful landmark for orthodontically customizing a mandibular dental arch form.
- The maxillary transverse skeletal dimension can be diagnosed by assessing a cusp-to-cusp distance of the upper posterior teeth relative to a fossa-to-fossa distance of the lower posterior teeth.
- The mandibular dental arch form serves as a template for the upper arch form. A coordinated upper arch wire should be placed only after a maxillary transverse skeletal discrepancy is corrected.
- A newer concept for assessing anteroposterior jaw position is "treatment planning to a smiling profile" using glabella vertical as an external landmark.
- The curve of Spee is often best leveled by tripoding the lower arch at surgery and leveling afterward.

Basic orthodontic principles integral for successful surgical rehabilitation of craniofacial malformations, cleft lip and palate, and more common developmental dentofacial deformities are fundamentally the same.

Depending on the specific cranio-maxillofacial condition, there may also be: clefting through the palate and alveolar ridge; associated palatal scarring and residual oro-nasal fistula; malformed, ectopic or congenitally missing teeth. In addition, characteristics of various malocclusions and abnormal jaw growth, unrelated to the primary disorder, are frequently present and often unrecognized.

Specific treatment objectives must address: the final occlusion, mandibular and maxillary arch form, anteroposterior (AP) jaw position, vertical jaw position, and chin prominence. Decisions regarding these 5 essential orofacial characteristics will influence the quality of general treatment outcome goals of maintaining or improving facial aesthetics, smile aesthetics, multiple orofacial functions, periodontal health, and both dental and jaw stability (Fig. 1).

From an orthodontist's perspective, there will be biologic boundaries to the safe movement (positioning) of teeth within the patient's available alveolar bone. If the biologic boundaries are not respected, periodontal sequelae (bone loss and gingival recession) and risk of dental relapse are high.

A comprehensive monograph on the topic of orthodontic care of each specific cranio-maxillofacial condition is beyond the scope of this manuscript.

[a] Department of Orthodontics, Medical University of South Carolina, 173 Ashley Avenue, BSB 347 MSC 507, Charleston, SC 29425, USA; [b] Plastic and Reconstructive Surgery & Pediatrics, Georgetown University, Washington, DC, USA; [c] Orthodontics, University of Maryland, Baltimore College of Dental Surgery, Baltimore, Maryland, USA; [d] Oral and Maxillofacial Surgery, Howard University College of Dentistry, Washington, DC, USA
* Corresponding author.
E-mail address: tremont@musc.edu

Oral Maxillofacial Surg Clin N Am 32 (2020) 321–338
https://doi.org/10.1016/j.coms.2020.01.006

## Treatment Goals

1. Facial Esthetics
2. Smile Esthetics
3. Function
4. Periodontium
5. Stability

Optimal or Compromise

## Treatment Objectives

1. Occlusion
2. Arch Form
3. Jaws AP
4. Jaws Vertical
5. Chin Prominence

**Fig. 1.** Flow chart demonstrating that decisions made regarding specific treatment objectives may be either optimal or an acceptable compromise, and will likely affect the outcome of any or all of the general treatment goals.

This article will focus on three specific orthodontic principles that apply to all conditions of jaw disharmony with associated malocclusion: 1) determining mandibular and maxillary dental arch forms, 2) achieving optimal anteroposterior jaw position, and 3) managing mandibular anterior height.

### MANDIBULAR DENTAL ARCH FORM

Optimal objectives for the position of mandibular anterior and posterior teeth require roots to be centrally housed within the alveolar ridge (for periodontal health) and crowns to be at an ideal inclination (for optimal interfacing with maxillary crowns) (**Fig. 2**).[1–10]

Using a patient's WALA ridge as a landmark provides a scientifically based approach to attaining a customized mandibular arch form.[3,5–8,10–13] The WALA ridge is a soft-tissue landmark just superior to the mucogingival junction and approximates vertically the center of resistance of the teeth (**Fig. 3**).[3,5]

The centers of the crowns' facial surfaces (FA points), when teeth are optimally positioned, bear distinct relationships to the WALA ridge (**Fig. 4**).[3,6,9,12,14,15] An arch wire shaped to the WALA ridge will therefore customize a patient's mandibular dental arch form primarily by tipping teeth (**Fig. 5**).

Because the center of resistance of the roots is generally centrally located in the alveolar ridges, buccal tipping forces to the teeth can biomechanically upright the mandibular posterior teeth to optimal inclinations while maintaining the roots within the alveolar housing.[5,16] Forces may be generated from expanded arch wires and/or progressive inclination twisted into the arch wires (**Fig. 6**). Mandibular incisor roots are optimally centered in the alveolar ridge at an average inclination of 75° to the occlusal plane (see **Fig. 2**).[1–3]

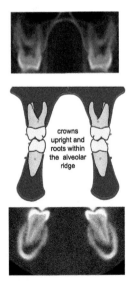
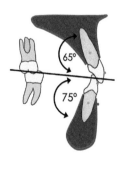

crowns upright and roots within the alveolar ridge

65°

75°

**Fig. 2.** Schematics, and accompanying cone-beam computed tomography (CBCT) images, demonstrating optimally positioned molars and incisor roots within the alveolar ridge and crowns at optimal inclinations. Blue dots depict FA points; red dots depict WALA ridge points; green dots depict tooth centers of resistance.

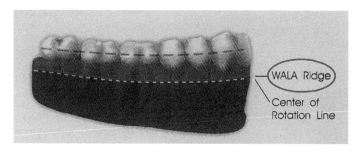

## MAXILLARY DENTAL ARCH FORM

As the mandible is not generally surgically widened and because the WALA ridge provides a reliable landmark, the mandibular dental arch form becomes a template for the maxillary dental arch form. A coordinated maxillary arch wire will, therefore, align the upper teeth to match the lower dental arch form (**Fig. 7**).[2]

However, it is essential to first diagnose the presence of any transverse maxillary skeletal discrepancy. With maxillary and mandibular posterior teeth optimally positioned (or planned to be optimally repositioned) within their respective alveolar ridges, comparison of the right-to-left side cusp-to-cusp distance of the upper posterior teeth (canines to second M) with the right-to-left side fossa-to-fossa distance of the lower posterior teeth can accurately diagnose the presence of a maxillary transverse skeletal discrepancy (**Fig. 8**A).[17,18] The calculation must take into consideration whether teeth in the arches need to be uprighted to optimal inclinations (**Fig. 8**B).

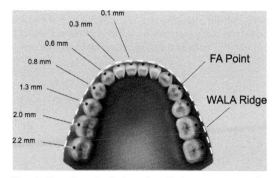

**Fig. 4.** Drawing depicting the distinct average relationship of the FA points of mandibular crowns to the WALA ridge from a study of orthodontically untreated optimal occlusions. (*From* Andrews LF. Andrews Journal of Orthodontics Orofacial Harmony. Winter; 2000. Permission to use this material has been granted by Lawrence F. Andrews. Copyright 2000 Lawrence F. Andrews. All Rights Reserved.)

It is critical to evaluate which upper teeth palatal cusps will occlude with which lower teeth fossae depending on the occlusal scheme (**Fig. 9**).[17,18] Also, there may be a difference in a given patient between the maxillary posterior transverse jaw discrepancy and the maxillary anterior transverse jaw discrepancy, particularly in patients with cleft palate, thus necessitating differential expansion (**Fig. 10**).[17,18]

Similar to the mandibular molars, the center of resistance of the maxillary molar roots is generally located centrally in the alveolar ridge. Palatal tipping forces to the teeth can biomechanically upright them to optimal inclinations while maintaining the roots within the alveolar housing (**Fig. 11**).[2,3,5,16]

When skeletally expanding the maxilla with a conventional rapid palatal expansion (RPE), miniscrew-assisted RPE (MARPE), or surgically assisted RPE (SARPE), tipping of the posterior teeth (usually palatal) to optimal inclinations should be performed after the skeletal expansion (**Fig. 12**A).[17,18] When skeletally expanding the maxilla with a segmented Le Fort I osteotomy, orthodontic uprighting of the maxillary posteriors should be performed before surgery (**Fig. 12**B).[17,18] This allows the surgeon to laterally expand the bony segments without rotating them to place the upper teeth into ideal occlusion with the lower teeth (**Fig. 13**).

It is critical that a coordinated upper arch wire should be placed only after correction of a maxillary skeletal transverse discrepancy by any method, or initially in the absence of a skeletal transverse discrepancy (**Fig. 14**A, C).[17,18] Before maxillary skeletal transverse expansion with a segmented Le Fort I, a narrow/constricted upper arch wire is appropriate to typically tip the posterior teeth palatally to an optimal inclination (**Fig. 14**B).[17,18] Following this discrete protocol avoids tipping crowns to abnormal inclinations, moving roots out of the alveolar process, and creating unstable tooth positions subject to relapse.

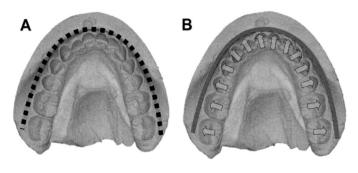

**Fig. 5.** (*A*) Photo of a mandibular cast demonstrating the WALA ridge (*dashed line*). (*B*) Customized mandibular arch form achieved by shaping an arch wire (*solid blue line*) to the WALA ridge. The arch wire will provide buccally directed forces (*green arrows*) to tip the teeth. (*Adapted from* Tremont TJ. Diagnosis and treatment planning for orthognathic surgery course manual. Cannonsburg, PA: Ortho Gnathics, LLC; 2019; with permission.)

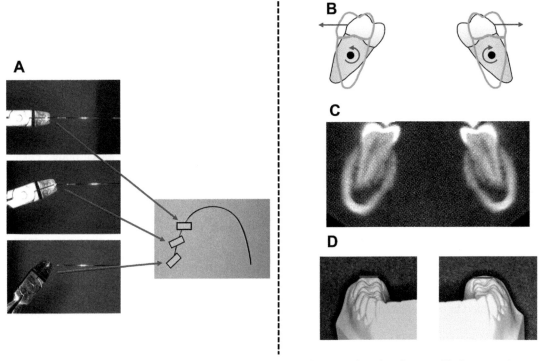

**Fig. 6.** (*A*) Image demonstrating progressive buccal directed inclination placed in the mandibular posterior section of an arch wire. (*B*) Schematic demonstrating a buccal directed force creating a moment to tip molars. (*C*) CBCT image showing well-centered and optimally inclined molars. (*D*) Photo of a cast showing optimally inclined molars indicated by their nearly level occlusal tables.

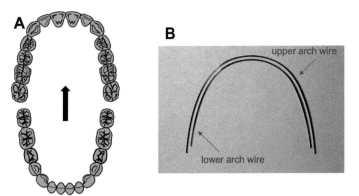

**Fig. 7.** (*A*) Schematic depicting a lower arch serving as a template for the upper arch form. (*B*) Photo of coordinated upper and lower arch wires.

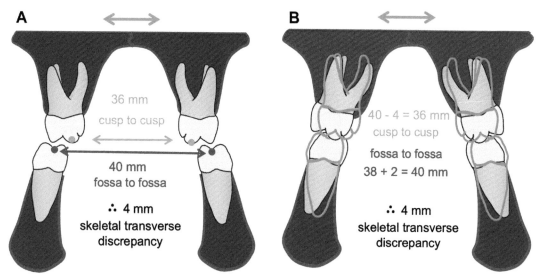

**Fig. 8.** Schematic demonstrating assessment of maxillary transverse dimension. (*A*) Cusp-to-cusp distance (*blue arrow*) between upright upper posterior teeth relative to the fossa-to-fossa distance (*red arrow*) of upright lower posterior teeth; skeletal expansion indicated (*green arrow*). (*B*) Calculation of cusp-to-cusp and fossa-to-fossa distances based on anticipated uprighted teeth (*green outlined teeth*). Note the absence of a posterior cross-bite before molar uprighting. (*Adapted from* Tremont TJ. Diagnosis and treatment planning for orthognathic surgery course manual. Cannonsburg, PA: Ortho Gnathics, LLC; 2019; with permission.)

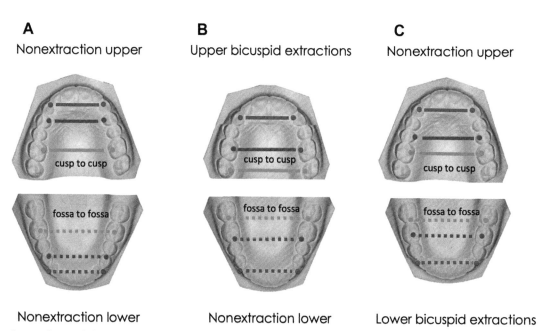

**Fig. 9.** Photo of dental casts demonstrating how to appropriately diagnose the maxillary transverse skeletal dimension. Upper posterior tooth cusps will interface with different lower tooth fossae in various schemes. (*A*) Nonextraction. (*B*) Upper bicuspid extractions. (*C*) Lower bicuspid extractions. (*Adapted from* Tremont TJ. Diagnosis and treatment planning for orthognathic surgery course manual. Cannonsburg, PA: Ortho Gnathics, LLC; 2019; with permission.)

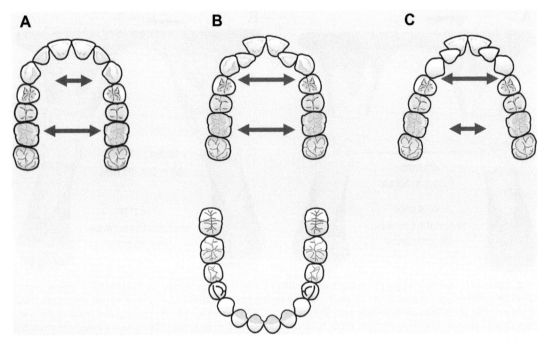

**Fig. 10.** Schematic illustrating 3 possible scenarios regarding maxillary skeletal transverse discrepancies. (*A*) Posterior maxilla needs more expansion than the anterior. (*B*) Posterior maxilla and anterior maxilla need equal expansion. (*C*) Anterior maxilla needs more expansion than the posterior. (*Adapted from* Tremont TJ. Diagnosis and treatment planning for orthognathic surgery course manual. Cannonsburg, PA: Ortho Gnathics, LLC; 2019; with permission.)

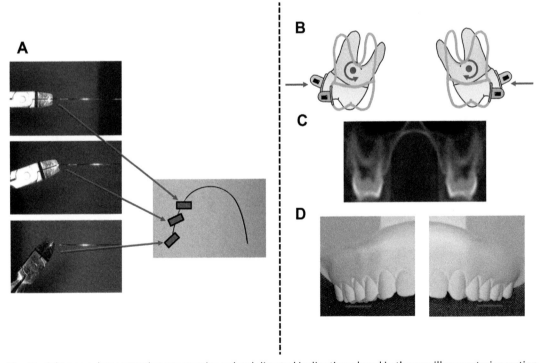

**Fig. 11.** (*A*) Image demonstrating progressive palatal directed inclination placed in the maxillary posterior section of an arch wire. (*B*) Schematic demonstrating a palatal directed force creating a moment to tip molars. (*C*) CBCT image showing well-centered and optimally inclined molars. (*D*) Photo of a cast demonstrating optimally inclined molars indicated by nearly level occlusal tables.

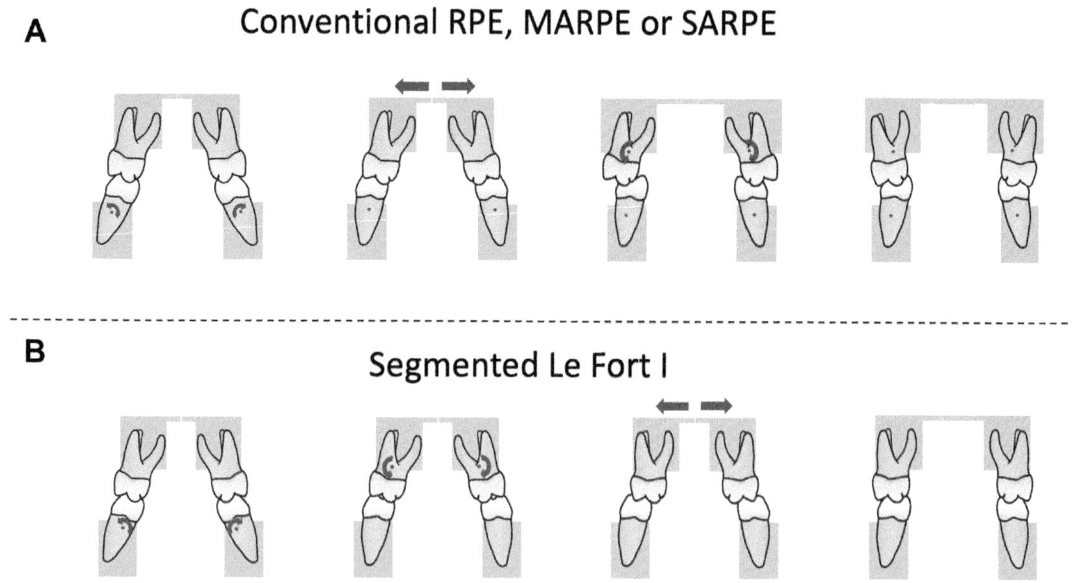

**A** ## Conventional RPE, MARPE or SARPE

**B** ## Segmented Le Fort I

**Fig. 12.** Schematics demonstrating when to upright posterior teeth if skeletally expanding the maxilla. (*A*) Maxillary posterior teeth are most effectively uprighted after skeletal expansion with a conventional RPE, MARPE, or SARPE. (*B*) Maxillary posterior teeth are most effectively uprighted before skeletal expansion with a segmented Le Fort I. (*Adapted from* Tremont TJ. Diagnosis and treatment planning for orthognathic surgery course manual. Cannonsburg, PA: Ortho Gnathics, LLC; 2019; with permission.)

Maxillary incisor roots are optimally positioned in the anterior one-third of the alveolar ridge at an ideal average inclination of 65° to the occlusal plane (see **Fig. 2**).[1–3] The effect on the posterior occlusion from coupling of upper and lower incisors with various combinations of inclinations is demonstrated in **Fig. 15**.[2,3,17–19] Understanding this concept allows the orthodontist and surgeon to anticipate final occlusions and, therefore, possible compromises to treatment outcomes.

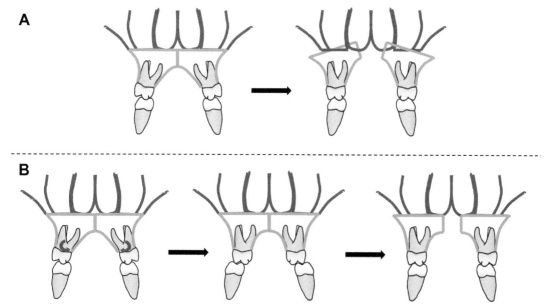

**Fig. 13.** Schematic demonstrating how: (*A*) buccally tipped upper posterior teeth necessitate rotating the bony segments to upright the crowns at surgery into an optimal occlusion with the lower crowns; (*B*) upper posterior crowns uprighted before surgery do not require rotation of the bony segments at surgery.

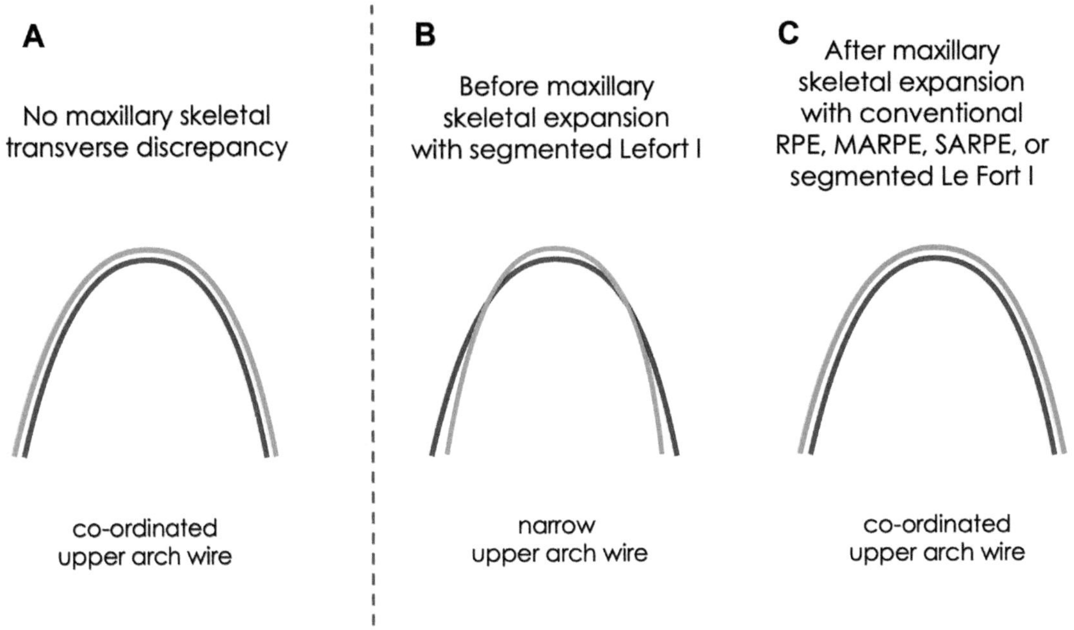

**A**

No maxillary skeletal
transverse discrepancy

**B**

Before maxillary
skeletal expansion
with segmented Lefort I

**C**

After maxillary
skeletal expansion
with conventional
RPE, MARPE, SARPE, or
segmented Le Fort I

co-ordinated
upper arch wire

narrow
upper arch wire

co-ordinated
upper arch wire

**Fig. 14.** Schematic demonstrating when to coordinate an upper arch wire with a lower arch wire. (*A*) Coordinated upper arch wires are placed from the beginning of treatment when no maxillary skeletal transverse discrepancy exists. (*B*) Before maxillary skeletal transverse expansion with a segmented Le Fort I, a narrow/constricted upper arch wire is appropriate to typically tip the posterior teeth palatally to an optimal inclination. (*C*) After maxillary skeletal expansion, with any method, a coordinated upper arch wire can be placed. (*Adapted from* Tremont TJ. Diagnosis and treatment planning for orthognathic surgery course manual. Cannonsburg, PA: Ortho Gnathics, LLC; 2019; with permission.)

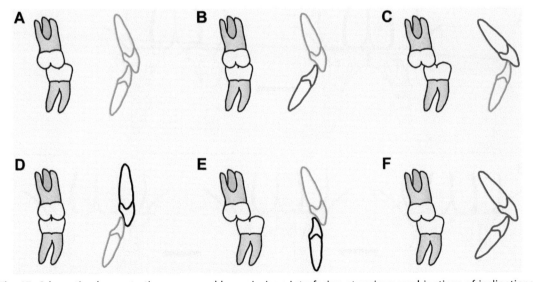

**Fig. 15.** Schematics demonstrating upper and lower incisors interfacing at various combinations of inclinations, resulting in different tendencies with the posterior occlusions. (*A*) Optimal upper and lower incisor inclinations with class I posterior occlusion tendency. (*B*) Proclined lower incisors with class II tendency. (*C*) Proclined upper incisors with class III tendency. (*D*) Retroclined upper incisors with class II tendency. (*E*) Retroclined lower incisors with class III tendency. (*F*) Equally proclined upper and lower incisors with class I tendency.

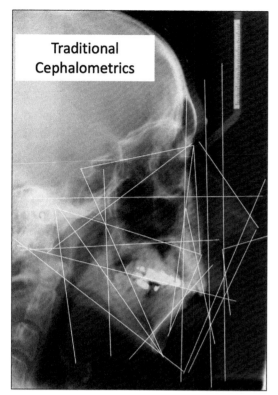

**Fig. 16.** Lateral cephalometric radiograph depicting various reference lines used in traditional analyses.

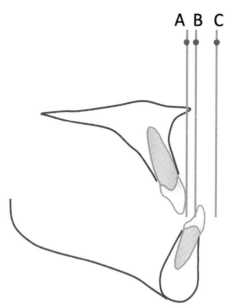

**Fig. 18.** Illustration demonstrating various hypothetical AP jaw positions. Glabella is indicated by red dot and glabella vertical by green line. Incisors are optimal within their jaws. A, orthognathic maxilla (upper incisor on glabella vertical) and prognathic mandible. B, deficient maxilla (upper incisor posterior to glabella vertical) and prognathic mandible. C, deficient maxilla (upper incisor posterior to glabella vertical) and orthognathic mandible.

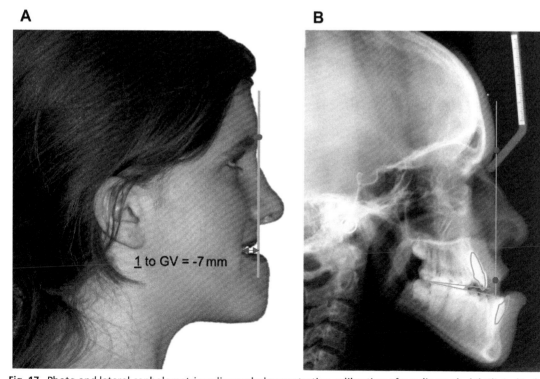

**Fig. 17.** Photo and lateral cephalometric radiograph demonstrating calibration of a radiograph. (*A*) Clinical judgment of −7 mm of the upper incisor to glabella with the patient's head in an adjusted "upright" natural head position. (*B*) Cephalograph calibration: a vertical green line (GV) is extended from glabella and 7 mm anterior to the upper incisor. Using optimally inclined and positioned upper and lower incisors (*green incisors*) within their respective jaws, this patient is diagnosed as having a deficient maxilla and prognathic mandible.

## ANTEROPOSTERIOR JAW POSITION

Traditional cephalometrics are abundant in measurements used in trying to qualify and quantify various dental and skeletal relationships including the AP position of the maxilla and mandible, and discrepancies between them (**Fig. 16**). However, landmarks such as S-N and Frankfort Horizontal are inherently unreliable because of their variability and broad standard deviations relative to norms.[20-39]

Andrews drew attention to evaluating the AP position of a maxillary incisor (optimally positioned within the maxilla and displayed when smiling) as a more accurate and reliable method for assessing AP maxillary jaw position.[3,40,41] Rapidly developing subsequent research indicates the usefulness of "treatment planning to a smiling profile" using glabella vertical (GV) as a landmark.[3,20,40-49] A preferred goal is to achieve optimal facial aesthetics with both repose and smiling profiles.

Using this approach, the patient's head is positioned in an adjusted natural or "upright" head posture and a judged measurement is made of the upper incisor to a visualized plumbed line tangent to soft-tissue glabella.[3,17,18,20,30-32,35,37,40-44] GV is a true vertical line representing a coronal facial plane. Transferring this clinical measurement to a lateral cephalometric image and planning an optimal maxillary incisor within the maxilla, provides a dependable method for discerning a realistic impression of jaw positions free of vague and/or misleading traditional assessments (**Fig. 17**).

In Caucasian males and females with an optimal AP maxilla, the incisor approaches but does not exceed GV.[3,20,40,41] A recent study showed that an optimal upper incisor/maxilla in African American females lies anterior to GV.[43]

Once the maxillary AP position is diagnosed, the mandibular AP position is also easily diagnosed by assessing the position of the optimal lower incisor to the optimal upper incisor, that is, overjet (**Fig. 18**). This analysis is particularly useful for diagnosing and treatment planning for cleft patients in whom the nasomaxillary complex is often significantly affected.[50]

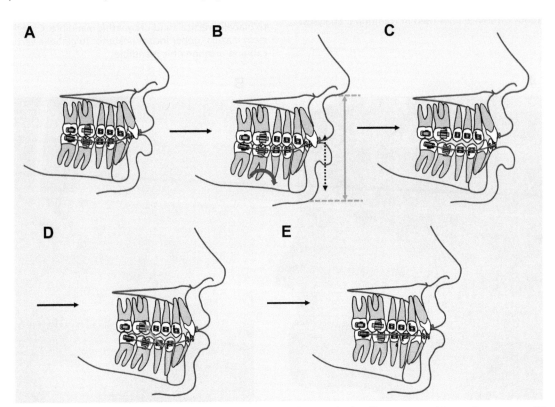

**Fig. 19.** Schematics demonstrating a reliable orthodontic technique for leveling a curve of Spee after surgery. (*A*) Class II deep bite with an excessive curve of Spee (*red* arch wire). (*B*) Short lower one-third facial height (*green arrow*), optimal mandibular incisor tip to menton (*dotted black line*), and planned mandibular advancement (*red curved arrow*). (*C*) Tripoded occlusion increasing lower one-third facial height. (*D*) Class III elastics to level curve of Spee posteriorly (*red arrow*). (*E*) Leveled lower arch. (*Adapted from* Tremont TJ. Diagnosis and treatment planning for orthognathic surgery course manual. Cannonsburg, PA: Ortho Gnathics, LLC; 2019; with permission.)

A              B              C

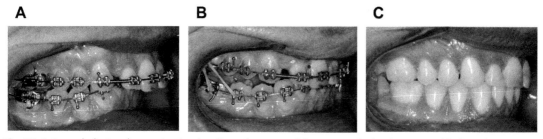

**Fig. 20.** Intraoral photos demonstrating leveling of a curve of Spee posteriorly after a mandibular advancement. (*A*) Class II deep bite with excessive curve of Spee. A 0.018 stainless-steel lower arch wire has a curve shaped into it to prevent incisor proclination from arch leveling. (*B*) Lower 0.012 niti arch wire in place after a mandibular advancement and tripoded occlusion. (*C*) Post-treatment level arch.

## MANDIBULAR ANTERIOR JAW HEIGHT

Managing orthodontically the vertical aspect of the lower arch form, that is, the curve of Spee, is critical to planning the mandibular anterior jaw height (incisor tip to bony menton) and directly affects vertically the soft-tissue lower third of the face (subnasale to soft-tissue menton). A lateral cephalometric prediction of a mandibular surgery (advancement or set-back) is necessary to access whether the mandibular anterior height should be increased or decreased (**Fig. 19**).[17,18]

If ideal to maintain the incisor-to-menton distance, it is often more effective and efficient to

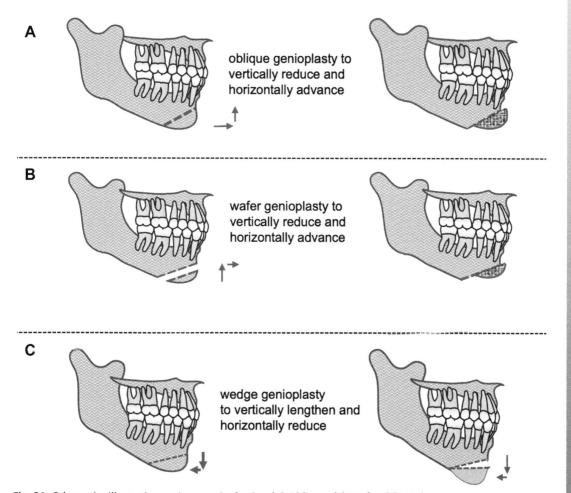

A    oblique genioplasty to vertically reduce and horizontally advance

B    wafer genioplasty to vertically reduce and horizontally advance

C    wedge genioplasty to vertically lengthen and horizontally reduce

**Fig. 21.** Schematics illustrating various genioplasties. (*A*) Oblique. (*B*) Wafer. (*C*) Wedge.

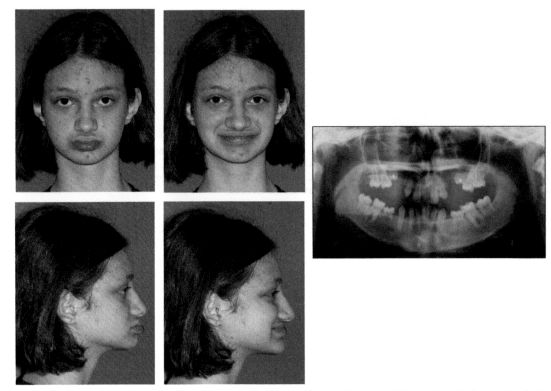

**Fig. 22.** Facial photos and panoramic radiograph of patient with symptoms consistent with ectodermal dysplasia. Note oligodontia, short lower facial one-third, and lack of tooth display on smiling.

level a curve of Spee after surgery. The lower arch is "tripoded" with the upper arch at surgery, and leveling is accomplished afterward using short class III elastics.[17]

Before surgery, a larger lower arch wire can be placed with a curve shaped into it matching the curve of Spee. This prevents premature leveling of the arch and excessive proclination of the lower

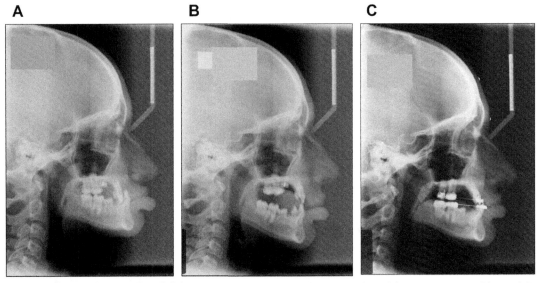

**Fig. 23.** Lateral cephalographs of: (*A*) pretreatment maximum intercuspation; (*B*) pretreatment with condyles seated; (*C*) presurgical with condyles seated.

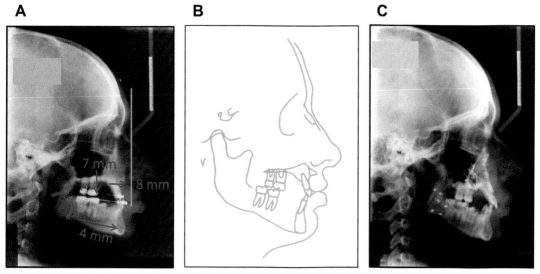

**Fig. 24.** Lateral cephalographs of: (*A*) presurgical cephalograph indicating a 7-mm maxillary downgraft, 8-mm maxillary advancement, and 4-mm mandibular advancement; (*B*) prediction tracing; (*C*) post-treatment cephalograph.

incisors. After surgery, a 0.012 niti arch wire is initially placed to allow for distal uprighting and eruption of the deep part of the curved lower arch with the force application for leveling coming from the elastic, not the arch wire. Using a light arch wire at this step prevents incisor proclination (**Fig. 20**).[17]

If the incisor-to-menton distance should ideally be shortened or lengthened to respectively reduce or increase the lower third of the face, this most often is effectively achieved with a genioplasty (**Fig. 21**).

## CLINICAL APPLICATION OF SELECTED ORTHODONTIC PRINCIPLES

Diagnosing and planning treatment of a patient's orofacial condition with condyles functionally seated in their fossae (centric relation) is essential for appropriate orthodontic and surgical management of both AP and vertical jaw positions, but also associated vertical aspects of the upper and lower arch forms (**Figs. 22–26**). In a vertically deficient patient, a seemingly prognathic mandible may actually require advancement when

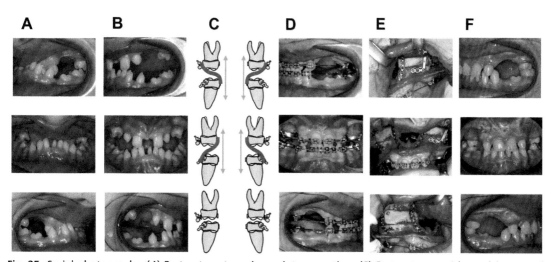

**Fig. 25.** Serial photographs. (*A*) Pretreatment maximum intercuspation. (*B*) Pretreatment with condyles seated. (*C*) Schematic demonstrating alternating cross-bite elastics. (*D*) Presurgical with condyles seated. (*E*) Intraoperative showing 7-mm iliac crest bone blocks. (*F*) Post-treatment occlusion.

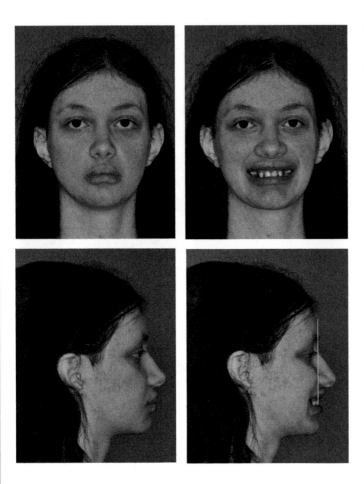

**Fig. 26.** Post-treatment facial photos. Note AP jaw positions, increased lower facial one-third, and AP and vertical smile display (Surgery was performed by Dr. Daniel W. Pituch and Dr. Richard E. Bauer).

accounting for seated condyles, advancement of the maxilla, and maxillary lengthening, which alone would result in rotation of the mandible down and back (see **Figs. 23** and **24**). In certain situations, upper and lower arch forms can be leveled presurgically by using expanded arch wires and alternating cross-bite elastics to avoid lingual collapse of the posterior teeth as they are erupted (see **Fig. 25**).

The transverse dimension of the maxilla is predictably deficient in cleft palate patients. Skeletal expansion of the segments with RPE in the mixed dentition can open the cleft site(s) prior to secondary alveolar grafting. Well-timed and successful grafting before canine eruption will provide necessary cancellous bone.

The required expansion depends on which upper teeth palatal cusps will occlude with which lower teeth fossae (see **Fig. 9**). Consideration, therefore, must be given when expanding the clefted maxilla to the presence of any maxillary AP jaw deficiency and the frequent absence of anterior teeth, commonly lateral incisors.

If planning to eventually advance the maxilla with a Le Fort I osteotomy, the upper dental arch will move forward to a narrowing portion of the lower arch. Therefore, an analysis must include quantifying the fossa-to-fossa distance of optimally inclined lower posterior teeth (adjusting for any planned uprighting, usually buccally) and quantifying the cusp-to-cusp distance of optimally inclined upper posterior teeth (adjusting for any planned uprighting, usually palatal) (see **Figs. 8** and **9**).[17]

With a deficient AP maxilla and missing upper lateral incisor(s), a segmented Le Fort I may be appropriate to advance the maxilla, close the cleft site(s), substitute canine, and finish with a class II posterior occlusion. The maxilla will likely need adequate expansion only to the extent for successful canine eruption in the mixed dentition (**Figs. 27** and **28**). However, more expansion may be required if a Le Fort I advancement, prosthetic lateral incisor, and a class I posterior occlusion is planned.

When a maxillary skeletal AP deficiency is not present and a segmented Le Fort I is not planned to close the cleft site, skeletal expansion of the maxilla must be sufficient to correct any transverse jaw discrepancy to open the cleft site(s) enough to

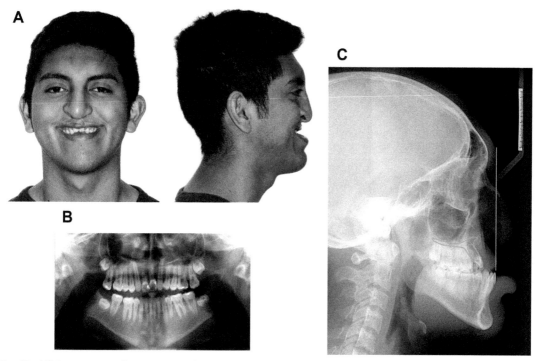

**Fig. 27.** (*A*) Pretreatment facial photos of teenager with unilateral cleft lip and palate. (*B*) Panoramic radiograph. (*C*) Lateral cephalograph indicating significantly deficient AP maxilla.

accommodate unerupted teeth or eventual prosthetic teeth (**Figs. 29** and **30**).

In the absence of a significant AP maxillary deficiency and a missing lateral(s), but with a limitation to rapid skeletal expansion caused by heavy palatal scarring and/or asymmetry, a segmented Le Fort I requiring less expansion can reposition the segment(s) mesially to close the cleft site(s) and finish class II with canine substitution.

The selected principles presented in this article will, it is hoped, provide the clinician with an initial sense of the importance of appropriate orthodontics for attaining successful treatment outcomes in cranio-maxillofacial patients, particularly cleft lip/palate patients. Optimal treatment objectives are often not attainable due to significant anatomic limitations. Nevertheless, the fundamental orthodontic principles discussed are necessary components of effective treatment planning.

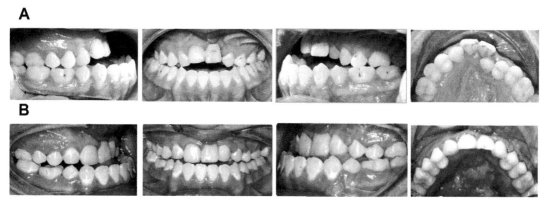

**Fig. 28.** (*A*) Pretreatment intraoral photos of patient in Fig. 27. (*B*) Maxilla expanded before surgery. Note that the amount of skeletal expansion provides adequate arch length for canine substitution, maxillary advancement, and a planned class II occlusion.

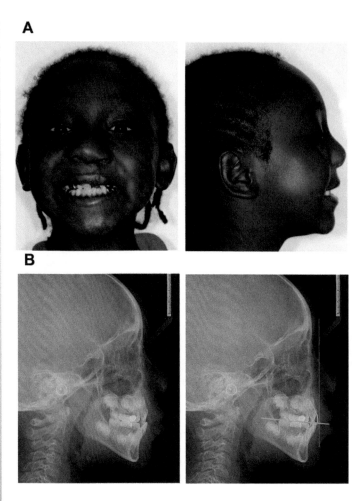

**Fig. 29.** (*A*) Pretreatment facial photos of a child with unilateral cleft lip and palate. (*B*) Lateral pretreatment cephalographs. Note optimally positioned coupled incisors indicating potential for class I occlusion; and upper incisor on glabella vertical indicating no skeletal AP dysplasia.

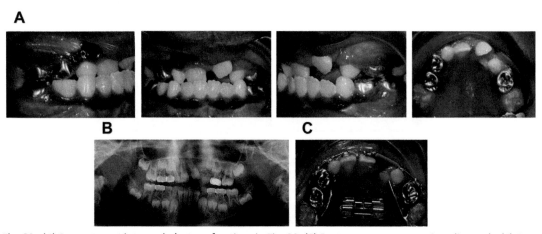

**Fig. 30.** (*A*) Pretreatment intraoral photos of patient in Fig. 29. (*B*) Pretreatment panoramic radiograph. (*C*) Post-RPE intraoral photo showing skeletal expansion prior to mixed dentition secondary bone grafting and adequate for anticipated prosthetic replacement of missing teeth.

## DISCLOSURE

The authors have nothing to disclose.

## REFERENCES

1. Andrews LF. The six keys to normal occlusion. Am J Orthod 1972;62(3):296–309.
2. Andrews LF. Straight wire: the concept and appliance. San Diego (CA): L.A. Wells Co.; 1989.
3. Andrews LF. Andrews Journal of Orthodontics and Orofacial HarmonyVol. 1. San Diego (CA): L.A. Wells Co.; 2000.
4. Bayome M, Park JH, Han SH, et al. Evaluation of dental and basal arch forms using cone-beam CT and 3D virtual models of normal occlusion. Aust Orthod J 2013;29(1):43–51.
5. Glass TR, Tremont TJ. A CBCT evaluation of root position in bone, long axis inclination and relationship to the WALA Ridge. Semin Orthod 2019;25(1): 24–35.
6. Gupta D, Miner RM, Arai K, et al. Comparison of the mandibular dental and basal arch forms in adults and children with Class I and Class II malocclusions. Am J Orthod Dentofacial Orthop 2010;138(1):10.e1-8 [discussion: 10–1].
7. Ronay V, Miner RM, Will LA, et al. Mandibular arch form: the relationship between dental and basal anatomy. Am J Orthod Dentofacial Orthop 2008; 134(3):430–8.
8. Suk KE, Park JH, Bayome M, et al. Comparison between dental and basal arch forms in normal occlusion and Class III malocclusions utilizing cone-beam computed tomography. Korean J Orthod 2013; 43(1):15–22.
9. Trivino T, Siqueira DF, Andrews WA. Evaluation of distances between the mandibular teeth and the alveolar process in Brazilians with normal occlusion. Am J Orthod Dentofacial Orthop 2010;137(3):308. e1-4 [discussion: 308–9].
10. Zou W, Jiang J, Xu T, et al. Relationship between mandibular dental and basal bone arch forms for severe skeletal Class III patients. Am J Orthod Dentofacial Orthop 2015;147(1):37–44.
11. Weaver K, Tremont TJ, Ngan P, et al. Changes in dental and basal archforms with preformed and customized archwires during orthodontic treatment. Orthod Waves 2012;71(45–50):45–50.
12. Ball RL, Miner RM, Will LA, et al. Comparison of dental and apical base arch forms in Class II Division 1 and Class I malocclusions. Am J Orthod Dentofacial Orthop 2010;138(1):41–50.
13. Koo YJ, Choi SH, Keum BT, et al. Maxillomandibular arch width differences at estimated centers of resistance: comparison between normal occlusion and skeletal Class III malocclusion. Korean J Orthod 2017;47(3):167–75.
14. Kong-Zarate CY, Carruitero MJ, Andrews WA. Distances between mandibular posterior teeth and the WALA ridge in Peruvians with normal occlusion. Dental Press J Orthod 2017;22(6):56–60.
15. Trivino T, Siqueira DF, Scanavini MA. A new concept of mandibular dental arch forms with normal occlusion. Am J Orthod Dentofacial Orthop 2008;133(1): 10.e15-22.
16. Smith RJ, Burstone CB. Mechanics of tooth movement. Am J Orthod Dentofacial Orthop 1984;85(4): 294–307.
17. Tremont TJ. Diagnosis and treatment planning for orthognathic surgery course manual. Charleston (SC): Ortho Gnathics, LLC; 2019.
18. Tremont TJ. Fundamentals of clinical orthodontics course manual. Charleston (SC): Ortho Gnathics, LLC; 2019.
19. Sangcharearn Y, Ho C. Maxillary incisor angulation and its effect on molar relationships. Angle Orthod 2007;77(2):221–5.
20. Tomblyn J. Facial planes as landmarks for diagnosis and treatment planning—thesis. Morgantown (WV): Department of Orthodontics, West Virginia University; 2015.
21. Arnett GW, Bergman RT. Facial keys to orthodontic diagnosis and treatment planning. Part I. Am J Orthod Dentofacial Orthop 1993;103(4):299–312.
22. Arnett GW, Bergman RT. Facial keys to orthodontic diagnosis and treatment planning. Part II. Am J Orthod Dentofacial Orthop 1993;103(5):395–411.
23. Arnett GW, Jelic JS, Kim J, et al. Soft tissue cephalometric analysis: diagnosis and treatment planning of dentofacial deformity. Am J Orthod Dentofacial Orthop 1999;116(3):239–53.
24. Barbera AL, Sampson WJ, Townsend GC. An evaluation of head position and craniofacial reference line variation. Homo 2009;60(1):1–28.
25. Contardo L, Ceschi M, Castaldo A, et al. Differences in skeletal Class II diagnosis using various cephalometric analyses. J Clin Orthod 2008;42(7):389–92.
26. Del Santo M Jr. Influence of occlusal plane inclination on ANB and Wits assessments of anteroposterior jaw relationships. Am J Orthod Dentofacial Orthop 2006;129(5):641–8.
27. Devereux L, Moles D, Cunningham SJ, et al. How important are lateral cephalometric radiographs in orthodontic treatment planning? Am J Orthod Dentofacial Orthop 2011;139(2):e175–81.
28. Durao AR, Alqerban A, Ferreira AP, et al. Influence of lateral cephalometric radiography in orthodontic diagnosis and treatment planning. Angle Orthod 2015;85(2):206–10.
29. Lundstrom A, Lundstrom F. The Frankfort horizontal as a basis for cephalometric analysis. Am J Orthod Dentofacial Orthop 1995;107(5):537–40.
30. Lundstrom A, Lundstrom F, Lebret LM, et al. Natural head position and natural head orientation: basic

considerations in cephalometric analysis and research. Eur J Orthod 1995;17(2):111–20.

31. Madsen DP, Sampson WJ, Townsend GC. Craniofacial reference plane variation and natural head position. Eur J Orthod 2008;30(5):532–40.

32. Moorrees CF. Natural head position—a revival. Am J Orthod Dentofacial Orthop 1994;105(5):512–3.

33. Naini FB. The Frankfort plane and head positioning in facial aesthetic analysis—the perpetuation of a myth. JAMA Facial Plast Surg 2013;15(5):333–4.

34. Pancherz H, Gokbuget K. The reliability of the Frankfort Horizontal in roentgenographic cephalometry. Eur J Orthod 1996;18(4):367–72.

35. Tian K, Li Q, Wang X, et al. Reproducibility of natural head position in normal Chinese people. Am J Orthod Dentofacial Orthop 2015;148(3):503–10.

36. Tremont TJ. An investigation of the variability between the optic plane and Frankfort horizontal. Am J Orthod 1980;78(2):192–200.

37. Weber DW, Fallis DW, Packer MD. Three-dimensional reproducibility of natural head position. Am J Orthod Dentofacial Orthop 2013;143(5):738–44.

38. Zebeib AM, Naini FB. Variability of the inclination of anatomic horizontal reference planes of the craniofacial complex in relation to the true horizontal line in orthognathic patients. Am J Orthod Dentofacial Orthop 2014;146(6):740–7.

39. Downs WB. Analysis of the dentofacial profile. Angle Orthod 1956;26(4):191–212.

40. Adams M, Andrews W, Tremont T, et al. Anteroposterior relationship of the maxillary central incisors to the forehead in adult white males. Orthodontics (Chic.) 2013;14(1):e2–9.

41. Andrews WA. AP relationship of the maxillary central incisors to the forehead in adult white females. Angle Orthod 2008;78(4):662–9.

42. Cao L, Zhang K, Bai D, et al. Effect of maxillary incisor labiolingual inclination and anteroposterior position on smiling profile esthetics. Angle Orthod 2011;81(1):121–9.

43. Gidaly MP, Tremont T, Lin CP, et al. Optimal anteroposterior position of the maxillary central incisors and its relationship to the forehead in adult African American females. Angle Orthod 2019;89(1):123–8.

44. Resnick CM, Kim S, Yorlets RR, et al. Evaluation of Andrews' analysis as a predictor of ideal sagittal maxillary positioning in orthognathic surgery. J Oral Maxillofac Surg 2018;76(10):2169–76.

45. Schlosser JB, Preston CB, Lampasso J. The effects of computer-aided anteroposterior maxillary incisor movement on ratings of facial attractiveness. Am J Orthod Dentofacial Orthop 2005;127(1):17–24.

46. Posnick JC, Makan S, Bostock D, et al. Primary maxillary deficiency dentofacial deformities: occlusion and facial aesthetic surgical outcomes. J Oral Maxillofac Surg 1982;76:1966–82.

47. Posnick JC, Egolum N, Tremont T. Primary mandibular deficiency dentofacial deformities: occlusion and facial aesthetic surgical outcomes. J Oral Maxillofac Surg 2018;76:2209. e1–2209.e15.

48. Posnick JC, Liu S, Tremont TJ. Long face dentofacial deformities: occlusion and facial aesthetic surgical outcomes. J Oral Maxillofac Surg 2018;76: 1291–308.

49. Posnick JC, Kinard BE, Singh N, et al. Short face dentofacial deformities: changes in social perceptions, facial esthetics, and occlusion after bimaxillary and chin orthognathic correction. J Craniofac Surg 2019. [Epub ahead of print].

50. Posnick JC, Kinard BE. Challenges in the successful reconstruction of cleft lip and palate: managing the naso-maxillary deformity in adolescence. Plast Reconstr Surg 2020;145.

# Moving?

## Make sure your subscription moves with you!

To notify us of your new address, find your **Clinics Account Number** (located on your mailing label above your name), and contact customer service at:

**Email: journalscustomerservice-usa@elsevier.com**

**800-654-2452** (subscribers in the U.S. & Canada)
**314-447-8871** (subscribers outside of the U.S. & Canada)

**Fax number: 314-447-8029**

**Elsevier Health Sciences Division**
**Subscription Customer Service**
**3251 Riverport Lane**
**Maryland Heights, MO 63043**

Printed and bound by CPI Group (UK) Ltd, Croydon, CR0 4YY

08/05/2025

01864746-0020